Rural Medicine

University Health Policy Consortium Series

In 1977, Boston University, Brandeis University, and the Massachusetts Institute of Technology established the University Health Policy Consortium to conduct health-policy analyses and research projects and to provide an educational laboratory for students interested in health policy. A year later, the Health Care Financing Administration designated the Consortium as its first Center for Health Policy Analysis and Research. The Center concentrates its research in three major health-care areas: long-term care, health-care quality and effectiveness, and regulation and reimbursement.

Brandeis University is the host institution for the Consortium, which is housed at the Florence Heller Graduate School for Advanced Studies in Social Welfare. Both the Center and the Consortium bring together social scientists, lawyers, and medical personnel to conduct collaborative research in health care.

This book represents some of the analyses that have been done by the Consortium's associates. Other books in the UHPC series are:

Reforming the Long-Term-Care System
Edited by James J. Callahan, Jr., and Stanley S. Wallack

Federal Health Programs
Edited by Stuart H. Altman and Harvey M. Sapolsky

Regional Variations in Hospital Use
Edited by David Rothberg

Rural Medicine

**Obstacles and Solutions
for Self-Sufficiency**

**Stanley S. Wallack
Sandra E. Kretz**
University Health Policy
Consortium

LexingtonBooks
D.C. Heath and Company
Lexington, Massachusetts
Toronto

Library of Congress Cataloging in Publication Data

Wallack, Stanley.
    Rural medicine.

    Bibliography: p.

    Includes index.
    1. Medicine, Rural—Practice—United States—Finance. 2. Rural health
services—United States—Utilization. 3. Federal aid to rural health
services—United States. I. Kretz, Sandra E. II. Title. [DNLM: 1. Rural
health—United States. 2. Rural population—United States. 3. Practice
management, Medical—Economics—United States. 4. Medically underserved
area—United States. WA 390 W195r]
R729.5.R87W34   362.1'0973   79-48057
ISBN 0-669-03691-9   AACR2

Published simultaneously in Canada

Printed in the United States of America

International Standard Book Number: 0-669-03691-9

Library of Congress Catalog Card Number: 79-48057

Contents

List of Figures
and Tables

Foreword

The improvement of ambulatory-care services in rural America has been high on the social agenda of people concerned with personal-health services for a number of years. Desires to revamp this sector of our medical-care system stem from the conviction that our current manner of providing medical care in rural communities is simply not meeting many health problems. Improved health, reduced disability from illness and disease, and increased family security are possible if we can provide ambulatory-care services more effectively. Likewise, considerable evidence exists that ambulatory-care services, properly structured, can reduce high-cost hospitalization expenses.

In an effort to improve this situation, several programs have been launched. These include neighborhood health centers, National Health Service Corps rural practices, "satellite" clinics sponsored by large existing hospitals and group medical practices, and nonprofit comprehensive rural health clinics.

The ideas that spawned these innovations have been with us for many years. However, they awaited the relatively fertile climate provided by the period between 1965-1980 for their introduction on a large-scale basis. During this fifteen-year time span, many of these ideas were translated into major national programs supported by a variety of public- and private-sector funding agencies, including the Robert Wood Johnson Foundation. These agencies hoped that through the funding of large-scale demonstration efforts, they could impress on the public the wisdom of investing in the development of these newer forms of delivering ambulatory services on a larger scale in rural America.

The sponsors of these different programs reasoned that after appropriate trial with national support, these rural demonstrations would find sufficient support locally to become financially independent. Given the rapid expansion that was occurring in the financing of health services throughout the country, it was hoped that national funds could be freed up and made available for revolving investment in new health-program development in other rural communities.

Unfortunately, these hopes were only partially fulfilled. The expectation that new rural health-care programs established in underserved areas could rapidly become financially "self-sufficient" proved to be premature. As a result, many of the most visible and important national efforts to improve front-line medical care in geographically isolated rural communities now find themselves in serious financial difficulty. The purpose of this book is to examine carefully this dilemma. What have been the factors that have so effectively constrained the movement toward major improvements in rural medicine in difficult areas of this country?

The Robert Wood Johnson Foundation is pleased to have been able to provide assistance for the preparation and publication of a study of this important question by the University Health Policy Consortium. It is clear from their findings, based on an analysis of case studies of individual medical practices, that the wave of new rural health programs predicted in earlier years will await changes of major significance in the way this country finances and organizes its ambulatory-care services in rural communities. Nevertheless, the findings do provide those who assist new practices with a better understanding of the necessary practice characteristics and implementation procedures that are involved in developing self-sufficient practices.

Robert J. Blendon, Sc.D.
Senior Vice President
The Robert Wood Johnson Foundation

Acknowledgments

In 1978, the Robert Wood Johnson Foundation funded the University Health Policy Consortium to conduct research on the financial viability of rural medical practices. Through the course of this study, Thomas Moloney of the Robert Wood Johnson Foundation provided insights and encouragement. Our advisory board members, Thomas Pyle, James Bernstein, Howard Newman, and John E. Ott, were helpful in the selection of the research strategy, the sites to be visited, and the major hypotheses to be tested. While the advisory board was extremely helpful to us throughout the research, we are solely responsible for the findings and the implications that have been drawn. We are most appreciative of all their support.

Charles Brecher and Maury Forman conducted a comparable study of urban practices. The sharing of findings and insights was useful.

This research could not have been conducted without the full cooperation of the physicians and other support personnel in the practices visited who gave us a considerable amount of their free time. The practitioners were open, frank, and thought-provoking.

A number of individuals at the University Health Policy Consortium, Brandeis University, also contributed to this book. The utilization data were organized and calculated by Marian Mitchell; Peter Leppanen compiled and analyzed the financial data; and Nancy Cannon contributed considerably to various aspects of the book. David E. Berman and Christine E. Bishop developed the linear programming model.

Stuart Altman, Sam Cordes, and Paul Gertman read and critiqued an earlier version. Their comments were valuable and contributed to the development of this final book.

Finally, the patience of Mary Smith and Mary Tess Crotty in typing the various drafts and of Katherine Raskin in providing editorial assistance is appreciated.

Rural Medicine

Introduction

The health-care resources of rural areas pale in comparison with those of urban areas. For the key health provider, physician differentials are especially large. There are approximately five times as many physicians per 100,000 people in cities with populations of more than 5 million than in towns with populations under 10,000. Since there are inadequate data on the other measures of medical underservice—health-care utilization and morbidity rates—the assumption has been that large differences in medical personnel, particularly physicians, result in large differences in access to health care.

Special programs at the local, state, and national levels have been developed to identify the physicians most likely to practice in rural areas, as well as to make the medical environment in rural areas more amenable to modern medical practice. While in the past it was relatively easy to construct buildings and provide equipment, it was more difficult to find physicians willing to practice in rural areas. As a solution, a number of new programs were created by the Department of Health and Human Services to provide medical workers and support services, for example, the National Health Service Corps, the Rural Health Initiative, and the Primary Care Research and Demonstration Program, formerly called the Health Underserved Rural Areas program. In addition, several other federal agencies (for example, the Appalachian Regional Commission, the Farmer's Home Administration, and the Small Business Administration), as well as major foundations (such as the Robert Wood Johnson Foundation and the Kellogg Foundation) and religious organizations, have become significantly involved in providing various types of funding and support to rural health programs. From modest beginnings, the national rural health effort has grown to involve billions of dollars and thousands of trained personnel in all categories of the health profession.

These efforts were founded initially on the assumption that rural populations residing in these communities would seek care at the new practices. With adequate patient volume it was further assumed that the practices would become self-sufficient after a few years. These assumptions have not been borne out, and requests for financial support have continued. Numerous studies have documented these phenomena. For example, in a recent study funded by the Appalachian Regional Commission, only one of the twenty-one medical sites studied reached the break-even point without outside funding (Swearingen, Schwartz, and Lee 1980).[1] The difficulties of achieving financial success in these rural practices, combined with the belief that these practices were crucial in providing access to care, have led to a shift in the policy objective from self-sufficiency to efficiency for the federally sponsored practices established in shortage areas.

If one believes that access is improved by these new practices and that they are providing care to local residents, one can reconcile the research findings of the difficulty of self-sufficiency with improved access by assuming that prices or fees in rural areas are too low to yield self-sufficient practices. This hypothesis, in fact, was the cornerstone for the research at the outset.

Purpose of the Book

This book was designed both to explore why financial self-sufficiency has been so difficult to achieve in rural areas identified as having a physician shortage and to identify socially acceptable solutions for overcoming the obstacles to self-sufficiency. While hypothesizing that lower charges or more free services (because of the preponderance of poorer populations) were causing inadequate practice revenues, we recognized that private, unsponsored practices existed in similar communities. Our strategy, unlike that of most other studies which focused on sponsored sites, was to compare similarly situated, sponsored and private practices. While we wanted to analyze the key factors determining average price—fee schedules, collection rates, and scope of services—it was decided that we should broaden the investigation to include the other determinants of financial self-sufficiency—patient volume and costs. Both have been discussed in previous research as obstacles to self-sufficiency, and our interest was in placing them in perspective vis-à-vis the average price.

These three determinants of financial self-sufficiency—the average price or charge per unit of service, the volume of services, and the costs to the provider of producing the services—in combination determine the net income of a practice. Since private practices continue to operate in rural areas, the charges of these practices must be high enough, given their total costs and volume of services, to yield a satisfactory net income (profit). Do they charge more than sponsored practices, operate more efficiently, or see more patients? Or is some combination of these factors working?

Of the three determinants, the individual physician, even assuming some monopoly power, has least control over charges or prices. Prices are determined in the general marketplace, and the physician, even if he or she is the only one in a community, cannot charge prices which are grossly disparate from those charged by other providers in nearby communities. In addition, third-party reimbursement rates of insurance companies often are based on the charges made by all the physicians in the geographic area. A private physician could see a different composition of the population, wealthier or better insured, and thereby raise the average charge or average collected charge, or provide a mix of services which yields a higher average charge. The private physician or sponsored practice has more control over costs. There are minimum costs in terms of space, equipment, and personnel, but both the quality and the level of the inputs can be varied.

It is in terms of the quantity (volume) of services, however, that it is often argued that physicians have the greatest latitude. As the patients' agents, doctors can significantly influence the medical services consumed. Of course, while the number and type of procedures performed can be influenced and hours of work varied, physicians have less control over whether individuals in the community will seek medical care for a particular ailment and whether they will use a particular provider when they do seek care. The conventional wisdom has been that financially successful rural practitioners encourage return visits, particularly for injections.

While the financial problems of rural practices have been extensively studied (Feldman, Deitz, and Brooks 1978; Nighswander 1977; General Accounting Office 1978; Holland et al. 1979; Rosenblatt and Moscovice 1978; U.S. Dept. of Health, Education and Welfare 1979), little research has focused on the interrelationship of the three factors contributing to self-sufficiency. Only Feldman, Deitz, and Brooks, in a 1978 study, concentrated directly on self-sufficiency, using original nationwide data. Rosenblatt and Moscovice studied the conversion to private practice of twenty National Health Service Corps (NHSC) sites in the Northwest. Others have considered issues related to self-sufficiency (such as utilization or costs) rather than total financial viability or have addressed financial self-sufficiency only tangentially. (Also data limitations constrained these studies. In particular, many of them used aggregate secondary data previously collected for another purpose.) Indeed, the significance of the three determinants of self-sufficiency—charges, volume, and cost—has been extrapolated from existing research since in no case has a study analyzed the three factors in combination.

Once the importance of the three factors in determining self-sufficiency is evaluated, policy changes which would foster self-sufficiency or increase the likelihood that a practice would become self-sufficient can be articulated. Our research has led us to consider and offer a number of policy directives. In developing these options, it was recognized that the pursuit of self-sufficiency may be at odds with two of society's other goals for the health-delivery system—quality and efficiency. The volume of services was found to be critical for self-sufficiency. In a fee-for-service system, the provision of *more* services by medical practices is encouraged. When this phenomenon motivates a practice to provide unnecessary services in order to achieve self-sufficiency, the tradeoffs to self-sufficiency are high-quality medical care and efficiency since more resources are being devoted to health care than are necessary. Because this project was limited to the collection and analysis of data on financial behavior, no attempt was made to measure the quality of health care provided in the medical practices studied. However, while quality-of-care performance is not a focus of this book, the policy strategies that emerge from our findings will consider the potential tradeoffs between practice self-sufficiency with quality medical care and efficiency.

The options developed for attaining self-sufficiency also recognize that adequate physician income is only one factor in determining whether a physician will remain in a rural community. It is, however, the one factor integral to the problem of practice viability which can be directly affected by health policy (unlike those such as preference for urban living and practicing near a university medical center).

Policy changes can influence the likelihood of financial independence of rural medical practices. Some of the reasons why new practices in rural areas have had great difficulty achieving financial independence seem uniquely related to their rural location. New practices are more likely to start in more urbanized areas, given the obstacles in rural areas of lower reimbursement rates and population scarcity. If policymakers want to equalize the probability of a new practice experiencing financial success in an urban or a rural area, changes in the reimbursement policies of federal programs as well as in the design and planning of sponsored practices need to be made.

The research findings are encouraging. While we have found severe obstacles to the development of financially self-sufficient rural practices, policy solutions are available. The problems and solutions for the practices studied are well documented in this book; however, the reader should be made aware that the case-specific approach adopted for this book does not allow us to generalize the findings and solutions to all rural practices. Although another study of similar number of practices may end up with very different findings, we think it is unlikely, since our findings are consistent with much of the published research on rural medical practices.

Organization of the Book

Because of the case-study approach we chose for this analysis, it is important to place our findings in the context of previous work. Chapters 2 and 3 attempt to provide this context. In chapter 2, the environment in which rural practices operate is described. Previous research has used a different definition of ruralness and access to care, and this chapter describes the rural environment and what data exist on access to care for rural residents. Chapter 3 moves from the general framework and issues to the particulars of previous research on the financial viability of rural medical practices, and in chapter 3 we argue for a research protocol that includes all the specifics of practice self-sufficiency—charges, volume, and costs—as well as original data collection.

The methods used in site selection and data collection are described in chapter 4. Since primary data were collected at very diverse sites, a number of accounting adjustments had to be undertaken to make the practice data consistent for comparative analysis.

Chapters 5 and 6 describe the financial findings. In chapter 5, the data on practices are presented according to the degree of financial self-sufficiency of the practices. In chapter 6, the financial characteristics and behaviors of the matched sponsored and unsponsored practices are considered. There is considerable overlap for practices between sponsorship and non-self-sufficiency, yet distinctions in the practices studied justify analyzing the financial data along these two dimensions. Chapter 5 considers all the financial determinants of self-sufficiency—price, volume, and costs. And chapter 6 focuses on costs and organizational arrangements.

Chapter 7 begins to describe why practice development, patient buildup, and diverse case mix appear to be very difficult for all rural practices, regardless of whether there is sponsorship. Having identified the importance of securing a high proportion of the population as patients for a rural practice and of performing a diversified range of services, the chapter goes on to describe why accomplishing these tasks is difficult.

Chapter 8 summarizes the major findings and describes the global as well as specific policy choices which need to be made. In considering the patient development problems that all the practices studied have confronted, it became clear that newly established practices must be both competitive and complementary with the rest of the health delivery system that serves the concerned rural population.

Practice development in an environment of competing choices and providers is a process that requires sensitivity and deft skills. If sponsored efforts are to succeed in establishing self-sufficient or efficient programs, then they must be structured for and continuously adapted to the environment in which they are located. Responsiveness must, therefore, be a criteria for any of the options adopted. By not building into their planning or developmental efforts the extent of the private delivery system, government or foundation programs reduce the likelihood of a sponsored practice becoming self-sufficient or efficient. Moreover, duplication in services and higher system costs could emerge.

Note

1. Medical sites studied included a variety of models, among them physician-extender practices.

2

Context of Rural Health Policy

Rural health-policy initiatives have been designed primarily to stimulate the supply of health-care resources in rural areas. The assumption guiding this policy is that a major rural health problem is lack of access to care because of an inappropriate distribution of resources—there are too few providers, and they are inaccessibly located. (These efforts to increase the supply of medical care are complementary to the major efforts to increase demand by poor and vulnerable groups through such programs as Medicaid, Medicare, and health education initiatives.) Programs that ensue from the rural health policy are targeted toward areas with concentrations of vulnerable people such as migrant workers, areas of high infant mortality, and the poor, which also have a documented shortage of medical providers. Because local projects are designed in cooperation with the communities, the projects are assumed to be sensitive to the nuances of the particular rural environments. Despite all these precautions, funded rural health programs have had great difficulty becoming financially viable. This chapter is intended to set the stage for the discussion of financial viability which follows, by presenting an overview of the rural environment and a short discussion of access to care in rural areas.

Changing Rural Environment of Health Programs

Because different definitions are used for the unit of measurement of "rural," often it is difficult to make comparisons or substantiate conclusions about rural problems. The 1970 census attempted to standardize the definition of rural, at least for use in government publications or analyses. Statistics are most often published according to two categorizations: (1) by a rural-urban dichotomy, with urban defined as all persons living in places of 2,500 or more that are incorporated as cities, villages, boroughs, and towns, but excluding persons living in the rural portions of extended cities; unincorporated places of 2,500 or more; and other territory included in urbanized (metropolitan) areas; with rural defined as all else; and (2) by a metropolitan-nonmetropolitan dichotomy

This chapter is a version of S.E. Kretz, "An Exploration of the Rural Health Paradigm: The Dilemma of Low Patient Usage of Sponsored Rural Physician Practices" (Ph.D. diss., Brandeis University, 1980), ch. 2.

with metropolitan defined as standard metropolitan statistical areas (SMSAs), a central city or twin cities with 50,000 persons or more, together with the contiguous, closely settled territory (urban fringe); and nonmetropolitan populations defined as all else. For both categorizations, often the rural and nonmetropolitan populations are broken down into farm and nonfarm, with the farm population defined according to the 1970 census as persons living on places of less than 10 acres with produce of more than $250 the year before or places of more than 10 acres with produce of more than $50 the year before and nonfarm defined as all else.

There are numerous problems with these definitions. First, there is often the temptation by researchers to use the terms *rural* and *nonmetropolitan* interchangeably, although the nonmetropolitan definition includes many places that rural persons consider "big" cities (with populations up to 50,000). Second, the rural population is not neatly broken down by place of residence—30 percent of rural people live in metropolitan counties (counties or sets of counties with a central city of 50,000 or more), and another 25 percent live in counties immediately adjacent to metropolitan counties (U.S. Bureau of the Census 1973). Thus, one must be quite careful about the assumptions made about rural people. For some 55 percent of the rural population, metropolitan services, including health and medical care, could be quite accessible, given modern methods of communication and transportation. Third, the rural-urban dichotomy does not give as clear-cut a picture of the population under discussion as one would like. Rural does not imply farm—less than 15 percent of the rural population live on farms, and of those who do, more income is obtained from nonagricultural sources than agricultural sources (U.S. Bureau of the Census 1974).

Finally, rural areas are not static, but in a state of change, with patterns developing that are not reflected in the 1970 census figures. Four major population trends provide this dynamic overlay to any statistics used throughout this book (Marshall 1976): (1) the continued displacement of persons out of agriculture; (2) the reversal in population migration between urban and rural areas since 1970; (3) the fact that manufacturing employment is growing faster in rural areas than in urban areas, although this trend is very uneven geographically; and (4) the persistence of rural poverty, which has not declined, but has increased since 1970, attributable to the high incidences of rural unemployment and to inflation.

Given all these limitations, this question might be asked: Is it possible to say anything useful about the health status of rural persons? National statistics, however, do show trends, and some patterns do emerge when population groups are compared on a rural-urban basis. These differences emerge because there are modal tendencies of the groups based on residence (Copp 1976). That is, although the rural population is not primarily agricultural, the agricultural population is found primarily within the rural population. Even though there is some variance in the income of rural people, a disproportionate segment of the rural population is low-income. There is variance also in the levels of educational attainment, but a disproportionate share of those with low educational levels live in rural areas. Differences also emerge because persons with great health needs (migrant farm workers, native Americans, and Appalachian whites, for example) are primarily rural people. With these data limitations fully taken into consideration, in the following section we briefly describe issues of access to care in rural areas.

Access to Health Care in Rural Areas

An assumption made about health care in rural areas is that rural persons have less access to care than their urban counterparts. A study of rural health care compiled by the U.S. Department of Agriculture (1974, p. 23) summarizes the position widely held in the field: ". . . one must conclude that rural and urban people do not have equal access to health care services. Rural areas are deficient in professional medical personnel, physical health care facilities, and the ability to afford the financial cost of illness." Discussions of access traditionally have centered on two issues: first, the presumed relationship between health status and access; second, equity—whether rural residents are getting their fair share of health services. The first has been historically the more prominent argument. In discussing the impetus for the funding of special health programs in rural areas, Sheps and Bachar (1980, p. 6) write: "Both the sponsors of these programs and the general public believe that the availability of an appropriate range of primary medical care has a direct effect upon the health status of rural residents." Access to care is also a central focus of discussions of equity. A summary of these arguments would be that not only do rural people have less access to care, but also governments have more of a responsibility to intervene to ensure access because rural areas are less able to compete for providers and facilities in the free market of health care.

Understanding access is fundamental to appreciating what national health policy, and especially health policy for rural areas, is all about. One problem, however, is the complexity of the concept. Is access a function of availability and convenience, that is, the physical location of providers and facilities? Is it associated with individual characteristics, for example, a lack of income to purchase care or of education about what "good" health standards are? How can access be measured—by utilization rates of health-care facilities, by demographic characteristics, by indicators of health status?

In their study of access to care, Aday and Anderson (1975) confronted the issue that access is conceptualized and measured in a number of ways.

Their extensive review of the relevant literature revealed that access has been discussed according to two themes:

1. The *process* theme derives from the assumption that the quality and quantity of an individual's passage through the health system are affected by the characteristics of the individual (age, sex, place of residence, and so on) or by characteristics of the delivery system (number of doctors, geographic dispersement, and so on).[1]
2. In the *outcome* theme, access is related to measurable outcomes of an individual's passage through the medical-care system, especially utilization rates and satisfaction scores. Proponents of this view argue that access needs to be examined according to external validations of whether those in need of care actually receive it.

For the purposes of this book, parts of the framework developed by Aday and Anderson are quite relevant:

1. Characteristics of the delivery system
     Physician resource distribution
     Effect of distance on access
2. Characteristics of the population at risk
     Extent of third-party insurance coverage
     Characteristics of the Medicare system which affect access
     Characteristics of the Medicaid system which affect access
3. Utilization of health services
     Gross measures of utilization volume
     Utilization in comparison to measures of need

This section uses the Aday and Anderson framework for considering the access problem of rural populations.

Characteristics of the Delivery System

In discussions of rural health-care access, it is the relative unavailability of physicians in rural as compared to urban areas that is most frequently mentioned. In fact, the concern over the availability of physicians is so predominent that it becomes virtually synonymous with access in many discussions (Kane, Dean, and Solomon 1978).

Probably the most commonly cited mode of illustrating physician shortages is the physician/population ratios by size of geographic areas (Way 1979).[2] Figure 2-1 illustrates that for total M.D.s involved in direct patient care, there are five times as many physicians per 100,000 population for cities of over 5 million (204) as for towns with population under 10,000 (41).

Physicians[a] per
100,000 Persons[b]

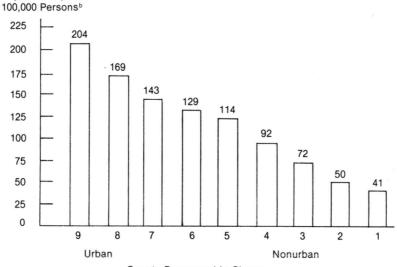

[a]Includes M.D.'s in graduate medical training.
[b]Resident population figures as of December 31, 1975.
[c]See chart below for the size of each demographic classification.

County Demographic Classification

County Size	County Class	Number of Counties
Nonurban counties with:		
Less than 10,000 inhabitants	1	769
10,000 to 24,999 inhabitants	2	907
25,000 to 49,999 inhabitants	3	484
50,000 or more inhabitants	4	229
Total Nonurban		2,389
Urban counties in SMSAs with:		
Potential metropolitan	5	51
50,000 to 499,999 inhabitants	6	330
500,000 to 999,999 inhabitants	7	128
1,000,000 to 4,999,999 inhabitants	8	170
5,000,000 or more inhabitants	9	16
Total Urban		695

Source: Louis J. Goodman, *Physician Distribution and Medical Licensure in the U.S., 1976,* Center for Health Services Research and Development (Chicago: American Medical Association, 1977). Reprinted with permission.

Figure 2-1. Nonfederal M.D.'s in Direct Patient Care per 100,000 Persons by County Size, December 31, 1976

In fact, there seems to be a direct relationship between the size of the county and the physician/population ratio.

This skew in the distribution of physicians is a phenomenon of the twentieth century resulting partly from the urbanization of the populations as a whole, the increasing sophistication of medicine and technology which is tied to a hospital-associated practice, and the increasing number of specialists who require a larger population base to support their practices (Brown 1974). Family and general practitioners are more likely than specialists to locate in rural areas. In 1973 rural communities had more general practitioners per 10,000 population than did metropolitan areas (2.7 per 10,000 compared to 2.3 per 10,000) (Kane, Dean, and Solomon 1978). The picture that emerges is quite different when the impact of specialists is added. When total numbers of physicians are considered, there were 6.7 physicians per 10,000 in rural areas compared with 15.2 per 10,000 in metropolitan areas, a difference of 127 percent. (There is evidence that specialists in internal medicine, pediatrics, general surgery, and obstetrics/gynecology are regular providers of primary care, and the number of family and general practitioners cannot be used as the measure of primary care available to the rural population.)

It is of particular concern, therefore, that an increasing proportion of physicians are specializing. From 1968 to 1976, the total number of nonfederal physicians active in patient care increased by 24 percent. Primary-care physicians increased 21 percent, while specialists increased 26 percent. More than half (53 percent) of all physicians in patient care were specialists in 1976 (Way 1979).

Another way of describing the rural-physician-shortage problem is in terms of the nonreplacement of physicians who die or retire in rural communities. The study by Hassinger et al. (1975) in Missouri demonstrated that the decline by 30 percent in the population of medical doctors and osteopaths between 1954 and 1973 was due primarily to death or retirement. Moreover, the decline could be expected to continue at its high rate because of the large number of elderly physicians still practicing in the communities. In 1973, twenty-six percent of the medical doctors and thirteen percent of the osteopaths were over sixty-five years of age; in addition, the percentage of both types of doctors under thirty-five was the lowest of any time in the twenty-year period.

The skewed distribution of physician services, however, is not in itself evidence of "maldistribution." Perhaps this urban-oriented distribution should be expected, given the primarily urban nature of the U.S. population, the large number of physicians engaged in teaching and research who are likely to be located in urban areas, the large population base needed to support some specialties, and the increasing emphasis placed on technology in medicine which, for the sake of economics of scale, is likely to concentrate physicians in urban areas.

Cordes examined this skewed physician distribution according to two criteria in order to determine if it constituted a barrier to access: the normative need of rural persons for more health care and opinions of physician-workforce experts on what should be ideal standards of physician availability. A normative need is assumed to exist when health could be enhanced by the production and consumption of additional physican services. On this criterion, Cordes (1976, p. 67) found that

> An abundance of indirect evidence suggests that a significant portion of the rural population faces a normative shortage of physician services. The literature, especially literature dealing with poverty, is replete with "horror stories" and statistical data on the lack of availability and accessibility of physician services to many rural people in need of those services. Among those most likely to be in need are migrant farm workers, and the mountain people of Appalachia.

To form the second criterion, Cordes examined five sources for standards of what constitutes good or desirable numbers of physicians per population.[3]

The findings and recommendations of all these sources are presented in table 2-1. The most conservative standard of 67 physicians per 100,000 population is still considerably higher than the actual ratio of physicians in the two most rural counties presented in figure 2-1 (counties less than 10,000 population had 41 physicians per 100,000, and counties with populations 10,000 to 24,999 had 50 physicians per 100,000 population). These counties comprised 1,676 of the nation's 3,084 counties, or 54.3 percent. If one used the more generous standards of physician ratios suggested by some of the other studies and recommendations, one would find an even higher ratio of the nation's counties falling below the standard.

Cordes concluded that based on the two criteria of normative need and objective standards, a significant number of rural persons face a shortage of physician services. That is, not only can one document the skewed distribution of physicians, but also, at least as demonstrated by national statistics, this distribution represented a barrier to access to care in some rural areas.

The second characteristic of the health-care delivery system identified by Aday and Anderson, which is of particular relevance to discussions of rural health, is the distribution of resources in the system, particularly the effect of distance on access. On one hand, it might seem obvious that the greater physical distances encountered by rural dwellers would constitute a barrier to access. Numerous studies, beginning with Lively and Beck in 1927, have noted a tendency of physician services to decrease with increasing distance of place of residence from the physician. On the other hand, more recent research has questioned conceptualizing distance solely as a function of physical space. In their extensive review of the historical development of the concept of distance in medical-services research, Shannon, Bashshur, and Metzner (1969, p. 155) conclude:

Due to problems of measurement, the total meaning of distance is not yet fully understood . . . the distance variable is only a crude surrogate for the human phenomena which are involved in travel. The measure of distance by mileage ignores the human attributes of travel. Certainly physical distance alone is not the true variable nor is it all we are looking for.

An example of the confounding findings in the research on distance and access is those of Bashshur, Shannon, and Metzner (1971) whose study of Cleveland, Ohio, revealed that only 6.4 percent of persons sampled in eight

Table 2-1
Suggested Number of Physicians per 100,000 Population

Name of Researcher or Recommending Agency	Criteria Used	Suggested Number
Schonfeld, Heston, and Falk	Provision of "good" primary care on basis of human need	133 primary-care physicians
Department of Health, Education, and Welfare (loan-forgiveness program for medical education)	Effective demand	67 total physicians
Paxton	Effective demand	50 general and family practitioners 20 internists 10 pediatricians 9 obstetricians/ gynecologists 10 general surgeons 89 primary-care physicians
Mason	Average physician/population ratios in six major prepaid medical groups. This ratio represents human need as expressed in the absence of price rationing.	16 family practitioners 23 internists 16 pediatricians 6 obstetricians/ gynecologists 10 general surgeons 71 primary-care physicians 94 total physicians
Stevens	Adjusted physician/population ratio in prepaid Kaiser Health Plan (Portland, Ore.). This ratio represents human need as expressed in the absence of price rationing.	71-93 total physicians

Source: S.M. Cordes, "Distribution of Physician Manpower," in E.W. Hassinger and L.R. Whiting, eds., *Rural Health Services: Organization, Delivery and Use* (Ames: Iowa State University Press, 1976), p. 69. Reprinted with permission.

sectors of the city utilized the nearest physician. Over 90 percent of those sampled traveled beyond the second-nearest physician to obtain care. Studies by Kane (1969) in Kentucky and by Kane et al. (1978) in Utah indicate that even though rural consumers have fewer choices in their sources of medical care, they are willing to travel considerable distances to obtain the desired care. At times they bypass more conveniently located providers, just as their urban counterparts.

Further, a study by Hassinger and Hobbs (1973) in four rural Ozark communities, with varying levels of health facilities available, found no differences among the communities in utilization of health services. Their findings led them to conclude that common normative standards of health behavior existed in the four communities which transcended the effect of physical distance—people sought care in situations where it was deemed necessary irrespective of distance.

Even though physical distance is, by itself, an inadequate measure of access, what can be said about the distance traveled to sources of care for rural people? Travel distance is often expressed in terms of time, since miles traveled for a consumer in the hollows of West Virginia may be not at all comparable to mileage for an Iowa farmer.

A nationwide survey by Aday, Anderson, and Fleming (1980) revealed that in 1976, as well as in a previous study by Aday and Anderson conducted in 1970, significantly fewer rural people had a physician close at hand (within 15 minutes' travel time) than did urban dwellers. What is even more interesting from table 2-2 is the changing patterns over time within rural areas. Access, as measured by travel time to a physician, improved from 1970 to 1976 for farm residents. The percentage of persons with a physician within 30 minutes' travel time increased by 10 percent, and most of the increase was among persons living within 15 minutes of care. Rural nonfarm residents, by contrast, experienced a decline of 9 percent for persons with care less than 15 minutes away and an increase of 6 percent in the 15- to 30-minute category. Using time traveled as the unit of measurement, one could conclude that as measured in the availability of physician services, rural persons have less access to care than urban residents.

Extent of Third-Party Insurance Coverage in Rural Areas

If understanding access is fundamental to understanding rural health policy, understanding the financing dynamics of health care is fundamental to understanding access. Davis (1973, p. 3) notes that the relationship of financing to access has virtually dominated the discussion of access in some quarters:

Table 2-2
Travel Time to Regular Source of Care, 1970 and 1976

| Travel Time | Rural | | | | Non-SMSA Urban | | SMSA | | | |
| | Farm | | Nonfarm | | | | Central City | | Other Urban | |
	1970	1976	1970	1976	1970	1976	1970	1976	1970	1976
Less than 15 minutes	21	27	44	35	70	69	51	50	58	51
15-30 minutes	54	58	45	51	23	26	40	43	34	42
30-60 minutes	21	13	10	11	6	4	8	6	7	6
More than 60 minutes	4	2	2	3	2	1	2	1	1	1

Source: Adapted from L. Aday, R. Anderson, and G. Fleming, *Health Care in the United States: Equitable for Whom?* (Beverly Hills, Calif.: Sage Publications, 1980), table 2.7, p. 58.

For some, access is strictly a financing phenomenon—and means simply assuring that medical care is not too expensive for individuals to obtain. Implicit in this is that many persons—particularly those with low incomes—will not purchase an "adequate" or "acceptable" level of medical care without some financial assistance.

Financing has been particularly prominent in the discussion of access to care in rural areas. There have been five main elements to the arguments:

1. Many rural persons are poor and have little money to spend on health care and health insurance.
2. More rural persons work in occupations where they are unlikely to be able to participate in less expensive group health-insurance programs.
3. Medicaid eligibility requirements do not respond to the typical situation of the rural poor where two-parent families are prevalent.
4. Predominantly rural states typically have the most meager Medicaid coverage.
5. Medicare reimbursements are typically lower in rural than in urban areas.

Davis and Marshall (1976) note that the lack of purchasing power because of low income is an important obstacle to the use of health services in rural areas. About 40 percent of the nation's poor live in rural areas, and the percentage of nonmetropolitan persons living in poverty is 14 percent as compared to 10 percent of those in metropolitan areas.

To explore the relationship of poverty to the purchase of medical care, Lane (1976) examined the "adequate package of health care services" defined by the Bureau of Labor Statistics for a family of four residing in urbanized places of 2,500 to 50,000 for 1971. This included a standard hospital and surgical insurance plan, plus services typically not covered by insurance such as physicians' visits and dental care. After examining the costs of medical care in relation to three budget standards (high, intermediate, and low), Lane found that about one-half the families in nonmetropolitan areas had annual incomes in 1971 below the intermediate budget and about two-thirds had incomes below the higher-cost budget. These families could have afforded the range of health-care services included in only the lower budget. Further, while the range of coverage in the lower-cost budget was more limited, it represented almost double the proportion of the family income (9.5 percent) as that for the high-level budget (5.2 percent). Thus, the poor rural families were sacrificing more to purchase less. Because the long-range growth of per capita income in rural areas has been less than the growth in medical-care costs, Lane conjectures that increasing proportions of the rural family budget will need to be spent on medical care.

These findings might lead one to assume that very few rural persons have health-care insurance of any type. This is not the case, according to the 1976 nationwide survey by Aday, Anderson, and Fleming (1980). Although this study did not explore the adequacy of coverage (that is, it is possible that rural respondents who said that they had insurance coverage had less than adequate coverage as defined by the Department of Labor study cited by Lane above), it is notable from table 2-3 that rural residents were only slightly overrepresented in the category of uninsured persons. Rural non-farm persons represented 20 percent of the total population, but were 22 percent of the uninsured population. Likewise, rural farm persons were 6 percent of the total U.S. population, but 8 percent of the uninsured group. The biggest differential between representation in the U.S. population and the uninsured group came from SMSA central-city dwellers who were 26 per-cent of the total U.S. population but 30 percent of the uninsured group. Most surprising is that rural dwellers were almost exactly proportionally represented among those having group coverage as they are in the total U.S. population.

The third element in the rural financing discussion is health coverage subsidized at public expense, especially for the rural poor through Medicaid. The major problem with Medicaid or rural-poor reasons is that eligibility is generally tied to state welfare eligibility, that is, primarily the aged poor, the disabled, and single-parent families. This has a particular

Table 2-3

Characteristics of People under Sixty-five Years of Age with Selected Modes of Insurance Coverage

Percentage Distribution of Demographic Characteristics	Group Policy	Individual Policy	Medicaid or Reduced-Price Care	Uninsured	Total Population
Percentage of total U.S. population in respective insurance-coverage categories	72	10	7	12	
SMSA, central city	24	22	39	30	26
SMSA, other urban	39	34	29	32	37
Non-SMSA Urban	12	10	11	9	12
Rural nonfarm	20	20	21	22	20
Rural farm	5	13	2	8	6
Total	100	100	100	100	100

Source: Adapted from: L. Aday, R. Anderson, and C.V. Fleming, *Health Care in the United States: Equitable for Whom?* (Beverly Hills, Calif.: Sage Publications, 1980), table 2.24.

Note: The percentage of U.S. population represented in this table equals 90; the percentage 65 years or older or not applicable equals 10.

impact on rural poor families which tend to have both parents at home. In 1974 over 70 percent of nonmetropolitan poor families had both parents in the home, as compared with 39 percent of central-city dwellers (U.S. Bureau of the Census 1976). The urban orientation of Medicaid eligibility leaves many poor rural families without coverage.

The impact of the urban bias of Medicaid can be illustrated through health-care expenditures as well as eligibility. Table 2-4 examines the proportion of the mean expenditures for personal health services for rural and urban poor persons in 1970. The public expenditures (Medicaid and other free care) for the urban poor are considerably higher. For example, Medicaid and other sources paid $76 per central-city child as compared to only $5 per poor rural child. For adults, Medicaid and other sources paid over three times as much as central-city individuals as for rural persons.

Table 2-4 also illustrates that urban persons spend more on health care, but a greater proportion of that is subsidized through public payments. Medicaid and other sources paid 75 percent of the expenditures for central-city children in 1970, but only 10.8 percent of the expenditures for rural children. Rural poor persons not only purchase less health care, but also have a smaller proportion of that expenditure subsidized at public expense.

A reason for the low rural Medicaid expenditures is not only that the eligibility requirements exclude many medically indigent rural persons, but also that Medicaid payments in predominantly rural states tend to be lower. A study by Davis (1976) compared the extent of Medicaid coverage, as well as the payment per poor individual, across the United States. There was wide variation in the amount paid per beneficiary as well as the extent of coverage for poor persons in each age group. For example, New York pays more than 300 percent of the national average payment per poor child, while three states pay less than 10 percent of the national average—Georgia, Mississippi, and Arkansas with less than $6 per poor child. On a national average, Medicaid covers 55 percent of poor children, while eleven states cover less than 20 percent of poor children—North Dakota, South Dakota, Virginia, South Carolina, Florida, Tennessee, Alabama, Mississippi, Arkansas, Louisiana, and Wyoming.

For the most part, per-recipient payments are substantially lower in the rural states than the national average. Rural states also tend to cover a smaller proportion of poor individuals. The results are almost universally lower Medicaid benefits per poor individual. The combined effects of more restrictive eligibility and lower payments per recipient make Medicaid coverage so problematic for the rural poor.

Medicare reimbursement rates are another key element in understanding the problems of rural health-care financing. They are important not only because rural areas tend to have relative large proportions of elderly residents, but also because the states tend to follow the Medicare lead in

Table 2-4
Mean Expenditure for All Personal-Health Services per Low-Income Person, by Source of Payment, Age, and Residence, 1970

Age	Total Mean Expenditures ($)			Medicaid and Other Free Care ($)			Percentage of Expenditures Paid by Medicaid or Free Care		
	Central City[a]	Other Urban	Rural	Central City[a]	Other Urban	Rural	Central City[a]	Other Urban	Rural
Low-income[b]									
Birth to 17	101	124	46	76	58	5	75.2	46.8	10.9
18-64	360	352	281	158	83	52	43.9	23.6	32.9
65 and over	446	329	407	54	38	27	12.1	11.6	6.6

Source: K. Davis, "Medicaid Payments and Utilization of Medical Services by the Poor," *Inquiry* 13 (June 1976):133. Reprinted with permission.
[a]SMSA.
[b]Low-income defined as family income below $6,000.

setting rates for Medicaid reimbursement (Sloan, Cromwell, and Mitchell 1978). That is, it is a federal requirement that Medicaid reimbursements cannot exceed those of Medicare for the same procedure.

The major concern with Medicare reimbursements has been the differential in rates paid to rural and urban physicians, as well as the implications of this for differences in physician income and the disincentive for physicians to locate in rural areas. The concern expressed by Davis and Marshall (1976, p. 7) is typical: "Even though coverage under Medicare may stimulate the demand by the elderly for additional medical services, the method of reimbursing physicians is not one which will serve to attract additional physicians to these areas."

A recent study by Burney et al. (1978) examined the Medicare rates on a national basis. These authors found that thirty-six of the states, representing about 95 percent of Medicare payments, differentiate allowable physician fees between urban and rural areas within the states. Another fourteen states, mainly smaller, rural states, do not differentiate between rural and urban fee schedules, but have generally lower reimbursement levels. This study of 1978 physician specialist fee schedules (the maximum fee allowable in the states under Medicare) revealed large differences among states and within states which differentiated rural and urban rates. On a weighted index, where the national average equaled 100, there was a difference of 173 percent between the highest county (Manhattan) with a score of 192 and the lowest county with a score of 70. On the average, however, the Medicare fees in metropolitan counties are 23 percent higher than the nonmetropolitan counties. When a cost-of-living differential is taken into consideration, metropolitan counties have fees averaging only 8 percent greater than nonmetropolitan counties. Burney et al. (1978, p. 1371) conclude, however, that this differential should not be minimized: ". . . after correcting for cost of living differences, Medicare payment practices provide financial incentives for physicians to locate in metropolitan areas."

Utilization of Health Services

Utilization of services is one of the two outcome elements of access identified by Aday and Anderson. (The other is patient satisfaction.) It represents the combining of the delivery system (supply) and the individual (demand) in a measurable unit which indicates whether health services have actually been experienced. Utilization can be measured in a number of different ways. This section presents utilization data according to both volume of physician contact and utilization in relation to need for services.

The use of physician services is one of the simplest indicators of utilization. Table 2-5 presents similar volume data from the 1970 and 1976 nation-

Table 2-5
Percentage of Persons Seeing a Physician and Mean Number of Physician Visits per Person-Year, by Residence, 1970 and 1976

| | Total United States | SMSA | | Non-SMSA | | |
| | | | | | Rural | |
		Central City	Other Urban	Urban	Nonfarm	Farm
Percentage of persons seeing a physician						
1976	76	77	78	73	75	68
1970	68	65	72	71	68	62
Mean number of physicians visits per person-year[a]						
Overall 1976	4.1	4.6	4.1	3.9	3.8	2.7
Those with one or more visits per year 1976	5.4	6.0	5.3	5.4	5.1	4.0

Source: Adapted from L. Aday and R. Anderson, *Development of Indices of Access to Medical Care* (Ann Arbor, Mich.: Health Administration Press, 1975), tables 9, 10; and L. Aday, R. Anderson, and G. Fleming, *Health Care in the U.S.: Equitable for Whom?* (Beverly Hills, Calif.: Sage Publications, 1980), tables 3.1, 3.4

[a]Trends for physician visits per year cannot be compared between 1970 and 1976 because of differences in the methodology of the two surveys.

wide surveys by Aday and Anderson (1975) and Aday, Anderson, and Fleming (1980). During that period, the number of persons seeing a physician generally increased. The biggest increase, however, was for central-city dwellers. Rural, nonfarm residents, who were at the national average in 1970, lagged behind by one percentage point in 1976. And while the visitation rate of farm residents increased during the period, it was 8 percent behind the national average in 1976 as compared to 6 percent in 1970.

Table 2-5 indicates that rural persons, both those who live on farms and nonfarm residents, saw a physician fewer times per person than the national average—3.8 and 2.7 times per year compared to 4.1 for the national population. However, the difference between rural and urban groups becomes less for those with one or more visits per year (a measure of return visits). Assessing this same trend in the 1970 data, Aday and Anderson (1975, p. 37) suggested:

> Some groups (especially non-whites, central city and rural residents, the poor and those with no regular source of care) delay longer in seeking the services of a physician. By the time they do see a doctor, however, the severity of their condition has probably increased, so that more visits to a physician are required to remedy it.

Aday and Anderson argue, however, that gross measures of utilization tell the researcher little in comparison to utilization measures which take into account some measures of disability. That is, Aday and Anderson (1975, p. 38) state: "Access to medical care is perhaps best considered in the context of whether people who need care receive it." Aday and Anderson developed a series of indexes for their 1970 survey which include measures of need as perceived by both the affected individuals (disability days, symptoms) and medical professionals (symptom severity and medical condition severity). Most of these indexes incorporate the concept of a use/disability ratio as introduced by the National Center for Health Services Research and Development. This is an attempt to integrate into one statistic any discrepancy between need in a population and the seeking of physician services in response to that need. The ratio is computed from the number of physician visits in two weeks per disability days (bed and restricted activity) in two weeks.

Table 2-6 presents utilization data from the Aday and Anderson survey by place of residence. Part A presents some basic data on whether people who experienced disability in the two-week reporting period saw a physician. It is interesting that even though there were rather noticeable differences between the urban and rural populations in those who saw a doctor during the year, these differences become much less among those who experienced a disabling health problem recently. Parts B and C of the table are helpful in interpreting this differential. Part B shows the use/disability ratio

Table 2-6
Utilization of Physician Services in Relation to Disability, by Place of Residence, 1970

	Total United States	SMSA		Non-SMSA		
					Rural	
		Central City	Other Urban	Urban	Nonfarm	Farm
A. Percentage with disability days in two weeks who had one or more physician visits in two weeks						
Yes	39	40	40	42	40	38
No	61	60	60	58	60	62
Total	100	100	100	100	100	100
B. Use/disability ratio (physician visits in two weeks per 100 disability days in two weeks)	14.41	15.29	15.66	14.70	12.52	12.26
C. Mean disability days for those with one or more disability days	5.41	5.56	5.30	4.83	5.51	5.79
D. Percentage with symptoms seeing a doctor						
Percentage seeing doctor as often or more often than they should	48	47	48	50	51	40
Percentage seeing doctor less often than they should	52	53	53	50	49	60
Total	100	100	100	100	100	100

Source: Adapted from L. Aday and R. Anderson, *Development of Indices of Access to Medical Care* (Ann Arbor, Mich.: Health Administration Press, 1975), tables 11, 12, 14, 15.

(physician visits in two weeks per 100 disability days in two weeks), which describes the volume of physician use relative to the number of days of limited activity experienced. The ratio for rural nonfarm people is 12.52, or 86 percent of the national average of 14.41 visits per 100 days of disability. Yet part C indicates that the mean number of disability days for rural nonfarm people is 102 percent of the national average. Rural nonfarm persons are slightly more ill (in terms of disability days), but experience fewer physician visits in response to that illness. Another interpretation of this finding is, however, that rural nonfarm people experience insignificantly more illness even though they use physician services at a rate 14 percent less than the national-average use/disability ratio, which suggests that urban dwellers may be overutilizing physican care.

Another need-based utilization measure presented by Aday and Anderson incorporates a comparison of actual use to the use level suggested for those symptoms by a panel of medical experts. Part D of table 2-6 presents data from the 1970 survey of those persons who saw a physician more or less often than a panel of medical experts thought they should, given their symptoms. It would seem that a discussion of access would include those who saw a physician less often than they should. Rural farm persons fare the least well in comparison to national averages. Some 60 percent of rural dwellers saw a physician less often than they should, a differential of 15 percent less than the national average of 52. On the other hand, the bulk of the rural population, represented by the rural nonfarm residents, fared better than the national average. Only 49 percent of these people saw a physician less frequently than they should in comparison to the national average of 52 percent.

Throughout the anlayses based on the work of Aday and Anderson, rural nonfarm dwellers were found to utilize physician services at about the same rate as the national average. It was the rural farm population (representing about 15 percent of rural persons) who consistently indicated less access to care as reflected in both overall utilization rates and utilization in comparison to extent of disability. This lack of utilization differentials by the vast majority of rural persons could lead to a number of interpretations: the use of gross rural-urban statistics tends to mask differences in utilization for vulnerable subgroups within the rural population, or the rural United States is becoming more like the urban United States in every way, including health-care utilization.

Conclusions about Access to Care in Rural Areas

The discussion of access to care yields a somewhat mixed picture. The framework for analysis contains three elements: characteristics of the delivery system (distribution of physicians and the effect of distance on access), characteristics of the population at risk (extent of third-party coverage of the effect of Medicaid and Medicare provisions on access) and utilization of services (gross utilization volume), and utilization in relation to need.

Given the rather large differences in the distribution of physicians between rural and urban areas and the fact that this disparity is often used to define a maldistribution and barrier to access, the findings in regard to utilization, even after adjusting for disability, are interesting. The rural nonfarm population is slightly more ill (in terms of disability days) than the national average (102 percent) and experiences 14 percent fewer physician visits, an amount much less than one would expect given the much lower physician population ratio in rural areas. On the other hand, rural farm residents seem to experience real differences in relation to both national levels of utilization and expected levels of utilization based on assessments of a panel of medical experts.

The findings about the influence of distance on access are inconclusive, partly because it has become recognized that distance is a complex concept incorporating more than spatial location. If distance is conceptualized as a function of time, rural persons do have less access. Again, the rural farm residents fared least well, but their access, in terms of more persons living within 30 minutes of their source of care, improved between the two national surveys in 1970 and 1976.

But provider distribution, distance, and utilization are only part of the total access schema. Differentials within public and private financing mechanisms still seem to constitute real barriers to access despite increased improvements in recent years. In particular, Medicaid payment schedules and eligibility criteria and the rural/urban Medicare reimbursement differentials are problematic.

The policy implications of these findings are interesting. The expressed demand for health care in rural areas (utilization per disability days) is much closer to national norms than one would expect, given the very large differentials in the supply of providers between urban and rural areas. One could conclude, then, that rural persons have become adept at overcoming certain barriers to access, especially those related to the supply of providers and distance. Serious demand barriers continue to exist, especially in the financing of public programs. Yet rural health policy has chosen to concentrate on increasing the supply of care available through programs which fund providers (both physicians and other types of health personnel) and facilities in designated rural areas.

Notes

1. It should be noted that some writers equate the availability of care with access. According to the Aday and Anderson (1975) framework, availability of care is only a small part of the access concept.

2. See the extensive review of the physician-to-population literature in Cordes 1976.

3. These standards were (1) levels of primary-care physicians per 100,000 population determined by Schonfeld, Heston, and Falk (1972), based on standards of what constituted "good" primary care; (2) standards of physician shortage determined by the U.S. Department of Health, Education, and Welfare (1974), which enable physicians practicing in such shortage areas to receive a "forgiveness" of some federal loan monies; (3) a study in *Medical Economics* (Paxton 1973) which estimated the number of physicians needed in various specialties to bring supply and demand into balance (only primary-care specialties are presented here); (4) the average physician/population ratios compiled by Mason (1972) for six prepaid medical groups; (5) and a study by Stevens (1971) of physician needs based on the experiences of the prepaid Kaiser Health Plan in Portland, Oregon.

Rural Health-Policy Responses

The preceding chapter examined the nature of the rural environment and discussed some of the elements of access to care as they pertain to rural peoples. If we assume that some government action is appropriate to meet the differentials in access identified, the major policy question becomes: what have been the program responses and have these responses been targeted at those segments of the rural population most in need? This chapter is divided into three parts: an examination of how much has been defined for program targeting, a brief description of the rural-health-program efforts, and a summary of previous rural health research, especially in regard to the financial viability of the programs.

Program Targeting through Need Identification

The cornerstone of federal methodology for the designation of program eligibility continues to be physician/population ratios, despite some evolution and increased sophistication over time. Basically, there are two methodologies. The first, which determines eligibility for the broad-based federal-funding programs, combines physician/population ratios with other sociomedical indicators to arrive at a composite Index of Medical Underservice (IMU) for Medically Underserved Areas (MUAs). The second, which determines eligibility for placement of physicians (and nurses, physician assistants, dentists, psychiatrists, optometrists, ophthalmologists, podiatrists, pharmacists, and veterinarians) under the National Health Service Corps, designates Health-Manpower-Shortage Areas (HMSAs) according to a formula which considers physician/population ratios with adjustments for factors of the service area and some sociomedical indicators. These methodologies and the programs to which they apply are summarized in table 3-1. Both methodologies have been object of some controversy.

The Index of Medical Underservice was developed at the University of Wisconsin, to respond to a directive in the Health Maintenance Organization Act of 1973 that priority be given to health maintenance organizations (HMOs) in areas designated as "medically underserved." However, not

This chapter is derived from S.E. Kretz, "An Exploration of the Rural Health Paradigm: The Dilemma of Low Patient Usage of Sponsored Rural Physician Practices," (Ph.D. diss., Brandeis University, 1980), ch. 3.

Table 3-1
Medical-Underservice-Designation Criteria

Designation	Number of Designations[a]	Criteria	Program Applicability
Medically underserved areas	7,519[b] (1,459 county 6,060 subcounty)	Index of medical underservice comprised of four variables: physician/population ratios infant mortality rate percentage of persons below poverty percent of population over 65	Rural Health Initiative (RHI) Health Underserved Rural Areas (HURA) program[d] Community Health Centers (CHCs)

Health-manpower-shortage areas	1,739[c]
	
	(870 county
	869 subcounty
		1. Rational service area
		2. Population/primary-care-physician ratio of 3500:1
		   or
		   population/primary-care-physician ratio of greater than 3000:1 and unusually high needs or insufficient capacity with current providers
		3. Contiguous-area providers are nonutilized, excessively distant, and inaccessible
			National Health Service Corps
			
			Loan-forgiveness program; scholarship support to students in the health professions who are then obligated to practice in shortage areas after graduation

[a]One is not able to determine the overlap between the listings for medically underserved areas and health-manpower-shortage areas. D. Zwick, "Health Systems Agencies and the Designation of Health Services Shortage Areas" Working paper, Robert Wood Johnson Foundation, 1980.
[b]As of June 1, 1980.
[c]As of June 30, 1980.
[d]HURA programs are now combined under the Primary Care Research and Demonstration Program, but are still referred to commonly as HURA in the field.

Congress, nor the Department of Health, Education, and Welfare, nor the Wisconsin researchers ever defined what "medically underserved" meant. As Wysong (1975) and Cordes and Lloyd (1979) point out, underservice could be interpreted as areas where services were not available or were not readily accessible, or where service-utilization rates were low, or where the outcome from service use was not acceptable. Instead, on the premise that it is presently impossible to directly relate changes in health status to changes in system components, an index was developed which could reliably predict how a panel of experts would judge the scarcity of health services in particular geographic areas. The index, which is composed of four weighted variables, was consistently able to explain more than 60 percent of the variance in the assessment of medical underservice made by local experts with knowledge of local conditions (Wysong 1975). In order of weight, these variables are the ratio of primary-care physicians to total population, infant mortality rate, the percentage of persons below the poverty rate, and the percentage of the population age sixty-five or older.

There is some rationale for the use of these indicators in addition to physician/population ratios. Lee (1979), for example, points out that the infant mortality rate may be used as an indicator of health status, the population over sixty-five as a predictor of increased health-services utilization, and the poverty rate as a measure of problems of economic access to care.

The designation criteria for MUAs have been criticized on four important grounds: (1) it is really a socioeconomic measure of a community, since extreme values on any of the nonphysician indicators could qualify an area as medically underserved, despite an abundant supply of physicians (Wysong 1975); (2) the IMU cannot predict differences in utilization or other important health indicators despite substantial sociodemographic differences in populations (Kleinman and Wilson 1977); (3) the typical unit for which IMU data are available (the county) is often too large or too small to make any judgments about adequacy of service to residents and medical-service patterns within the county or in contiguous counties; and (4) in order to designate subcounty shortage areas, data from two of the indicators (physician/population ratio and infant mortality), which are available on a county basis, are combined with other indicators (poverty and aged) that are available for census tracts or civil divisions.

The concept of a health manpower shortage is narrower than that of medical underservice—it is directed at the problems of inadequate care resulting from a lack of medical personnel, whereas the IMU pertains to inadequate care for any number of reasons.

Begun in 1965, the manpower-shortage designation process was first used as part of a loan-forgiveness program (Lee 1979). The 1972 amendments to the NHSC legislation brought increased attraction to the issue by requiring that NHSC personnel be placed in "critical health manpower shortage areas," which were determined in a relatively straightforward way of a physician/population ratio of 1/4,000 on a county or subcounty level. The heavy reliance on the physician/population ratios tended to obscure local differences in health needs, in demands for care, in levels of physician productivity, and in the presence of other health-care resources which augment providers (Lee 1979). In 1976 the Health Professions Education Assistance Act required that new criteria supplement provider/population ratios with concepts of rational service areas, indicators of need for health services, and a method of prioritizing shortage areas. An important additional change was the authority to designate particular population groups or facilities as shortage "areas" (for example, federal prisons) as well as geographic areas.

The new criteria, which became effective in 1978, designate shortage areas separately for different types of medical workforce.[1] The manpower shortage areas for primary care have been the principal focus of rural health policy, and they are illustrated in figure 3-1.

For each of the seven types of health manpower, the three considerations (rational service areas, within-area criteria, and contiguous-area criteria) are applied somewhat differently (Lee 1979).[2] For example, a rational service area is defined as 30 minutes' travel time for primary care and 40 minutes' for dental care. The within-area criteria still use provider/population ratios as the main indicator, but these are modified for each type of health manpower as well as supplemented with other indicators. The designation for primary care of 3,500:1 represents about 150 percent of the median U.S. county ratios.

The other indicators of high need especially help to highlight urban shortage areas. Status measures such as high infant mortality, high fertility rates, and large incidences of poverty are used as well as use indicators such as excessive waiting times and excessive numbers of visits per year to existing full-time primary-care physicians. The contiguous-area criteria, which must be considered before an HMSA is designated, attempt to explore if other health resources could affect a potential shortage area: whether the contiguous-area manpower is beyond the excessive travel limit and is thus inaccessible; whether the contiguous-area provider/population ratios are above a certain level, indicating these practitioners would be unavailable to relieve the excess demand of the shortage area; and whether some other access barriers prevent persons in the potential HMSA from using health resources in the contiguous areas.

Although the new HMSA designation criteria do much to eliminate the problems of the previous methodology, a number of concerns remain (Rosenblatt and Moscovice 1980):

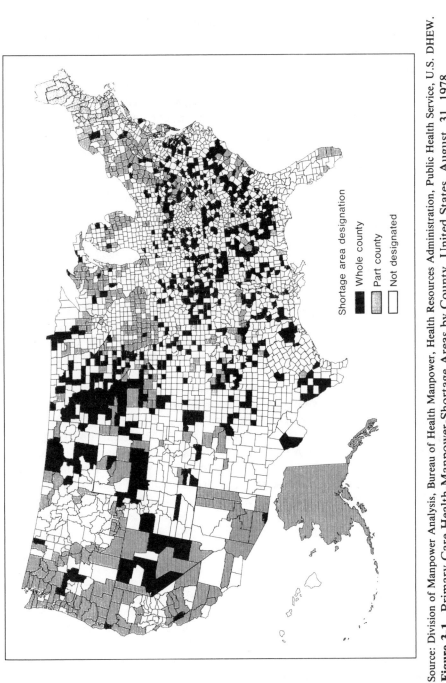

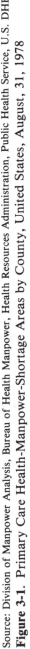

Source: Division of Manpower Analysis, Bureau of Health Manpower, Health Resources Administration, Public Health Service, U.S. DHEW.

Figure 3-1. Primary Care Health-Manpower-Shortage Areas by County, United States, August, 31, 1978

1. The new flexibility to designate institutions and population groups as HMSAs makes it more difficult to project future manpower needs—theoretically, almost an unlimited number of "areas" could be designated.
2. The lack of a ceiling on manpower "need" is at least partially related to the fact that the number of scholarships has been a function of congressional appropriations rather than an attempt to field a certain percentage of the calculated needed physicians in rural areas.
3. HMSA designations are still dependent on a data collected on a geopolitical basis, even though these may bear no relationship to medical-service areas.
4. There is little agreement on which population characteristics are the most important indicators of need and should be used to supplement provider/population ratios in designating HMSAs. Hence there is still the primary reliance on provider/population ratios.

It is clear from the discussion of shortage-area designation that despite a great deal of effort, current methods for measuring the additional quality of health services needed (by using MUA and HMSA criteria) are far from satisfactory. This is especially so since they rely on indicators of supply and need and do not examine local utilization rates. As noted in chapter 2, utilization is much closer to the national norms than would be expected, given the large differentials in supply and need.

As is frequently true in matters of public policy, however, programmatic responses are required despite inadequate knowledge. Whatever the shortcomings of the current method of targeting program efforts, they reflect an assumption that current health care in these areas is sufficiently inadequate to warrant governmental intervention. The designation criteria are in actuality a screening device for possible areas requiring program targeting. That they are not completely accurate makes program development at the local level even more crucial. The next section briefly describes the major rural health programs which respond to these assumptions of inadequate supply of care.

Program Responses in Rural Health

In this section we discuss six major rural health programs: the National Health Service Corps (NHSC), the Rural Health Initiative (RHI), the Community Health Centers (CHC) program, the Health Underserved Rural Areas (HURA) program, the Migrant Health Centers programs, and the Appalachian health programs.[3] The federal strategy has two major components. The first is an emphasis on manpower, and the second is program development—the encouragement of comprehensive planning, the development of innovative service-delivery mechanisms, and the support of health-care services to particular, designated service areas. As in many other areas, there is not a neat division of program thrusts—manpower supported under the National Health Service Corps is often used as a component to other federally funded programs.

The cornerstone of federal rural health policy has become the National Health Service Corps, which developed in local communities both as an independent program and as a manpower source for other funded programs, such as HURA and CHC. Recent NHSC policy has emphasized multiprovider placements and a more comprehensive approach to planning and programming, in contrast to the independent solo-physician sites often developed in the early years of the program.

The NHSC "program" has two separate thrusts. The first is the provision of health manpower. The NHSC fields seven different types of manpower, although the overwhelming majority has always been physicians. The second major thrust is a financial-aid component which provides scholarships to students who are committed to serve in the NHSC after completing their education (or who must repay the scholarship plus a penalty). In 1976 the Health Professions Educational Assistance Act significantly expanded the scholarship program with an appropriation greater than that for field operations. Rosenblatt and Moscovice (1980) note that the NHSC scholarship program has become the government's major vehicle for financing medical-student scholarships, and they suggest that the link to eventual field service results more from a philosophy that medical personnel should serve to help pay for their educations than from a community-based assessment for a specific number of medical professionals to respond to unmet health needs.

The NHSC has gone through four major programmatic shifts since its inception, all interrelated. The first is an emphasis on the short-term goal of providing medical manpower to underserved areas, away from original program conceptions that a substantial number of providers would remain in their communities as private physicians (Redman 1973); General Accounting Office 1978; Rosenblatt and Moscovice 1980). Second, related to the first is the shift to a goal of efficient service provision and away from the goal of financial self-sufficiency (Cordes and Lloyd 1979). Third, there is a movement away from the solo-private-physician model to incorporation of physician manpower into more comprehensive programs, including preventive services, which are not expected to be self-supporting (Rosenblatt and Moscovice 1980; General Accounting Office 1978). Fourth, there is an increased commitment of program resources, projected at about 15 percent for fiscal year 1979, to urban programs (Ahearn 1979).

The Rural Health Initiative (RHI) is not a legislatively established program. Rather, it is an administrative effort to coordinate and integrate a number of existing health programs in rural areas: the CHC program, the NHSC program, the HURA program, and the Migrant and Appalachian health programs. As discussed by Ahearn, these programs operated independently before the initiation of RHI and could have served the same population or community with separate efforts and facilities. A major purpose of RHI is to convert such narrowly based program efforts to comprehensive and coordinated health-care programs. RHI uses its funds to support programs which also have other rural-health-program components. For example, over half of the RHI projects are also designated HMSAs to receive manpower support from NHSC. There is also an effort to coordinate programming with the Area Health Education Center (AHEC) projects of the Health Resources Administration; the Drug Abuse Program of the Alcohol, Drug, and Mental Health Administration; Cervical Cytology Clinics and Breast Cancer Detection programs of the National Institutes of Health; and the Women, Infants, and Children (WIC) program of the Department of Agriculture, which is concerned with nutrition and food supplements (Kane, Dean, and Solomon 1978).

A program with a traditionally urban focus, which is now becoming more sensitive to rural needs, is that of the Community Health Centers (CHCs). This program has combined several different program thrusts. The largest component, the OEO Neighborhood Health Centers, began under the Office of Economic Opportunity (OEO) legislation in 1964 . Other programs include: the Neighborhood Health Centers (NHC), authorized under section 314(e) of the Comprehensive Health Planning and Public Health Services Act of 1966; the Community Health Networks (CHNs), and Family Health Centers (FHCs), which are prepaid capitation programs for ambulatory care. In fiscal year 1978, about 80 percent of CHC funding was still devoted to programs operating in the model of the early NHC—large, comprehensive programs, which often have diverse goals, such as employment of neighborhood persons and development of career ladders for the poor, and little focus on financial self-sufficiency. The high costs of these programs, plus the traditional urban orientation of the OEO programs, left little room for new rural programs without substantial increases in total program funding. In fiscal year 1978, only about 20 percent of CHC program users were rural people (Ahearn 1979). In fiscal year 1979, the Department of Health, Education, and Welfare (DHEW) instituted new requirements for giving rural persons a larger share of the new-users slots, which should have some effect over time.

The Health Underserved Rural Areas (HURA) program began in response to a Senate Appropriations Committee directive (Committee Report No. 93-1146) for the formation of a rural health research and demonstration program, in late 1974. It was originally established under the research and demonstration authority and section 1110 of the Social Security Act, and it was administered by the Medical Services Administration of the Social and Rehabilitation Services. Since 1976, it has been administered by the Office of Rural Health in the Bureau of Community Health Services, Public Health Service. Funds are used for the demonstration of research on primary health or dental care. Especially relevant are projects that demonstrate unique and innovative delivery systems or demonstrate methods of attracting health personnel or providing services. A cornerstone of the HURA program is the assumption that improved patient outcome and reduced costs result from improved methods of health care—from efficient resource allocation and management (Kane, Dean, and Solomon 1978).

In 1978 the Primary Care Research and Demonstration Program was established under section 340 of the Public Health Service Act, which would have expanded and revised the HURA authority. No funds were appropriated for projects under this program. The program has continued to operate on a limited scale under section 1110 authority, with some local projects transferred to the RHI program.

The Migrant Health Centers program has evolved over time since the early 1960s when authority for migrant programs was divided between HEW and OEO. The authority for migrant health programs traces to a 1962 law, the Migrant Health Act, which was amended numerous times before emerging as a new authority in Title IV of the Health Revenue Sharing and Health Services Act of 1975. An aspect of that law is to require that programs be located in high-impact areas (areas designated by the Migrant Health Services, Bureau of Community Health Services, as having at least 4,000 migrants and/or seasonal farm workers and their families for at least two months of the year). The act also specifies more clearly what a migrant health center is and authorizes grants to public and private nonprofit bodies to plan, initiate, and conduct local migrant health programs. The goal of the Migrant Health Centers program is to promote the provision of quality health-care services through the provision of diagnostic, treatment, and preventive services. Additional services such as dental care, health and nutrition counseling, and environmental services may be provided as well (Ahearn 1979).

The Appalachian health program was authorized by section 202 of the Appalachian Development Act "in order to demonstrate the value of adequate health facilities and services to the economic development of the Region." It provided for the construction and operation of hospitals and other health facilities within the Appalachian region, which covers parts of thirteen states. The overall goals of the Appalachian health program are to improve the health status of persons in the region, improve access to care, and reduce cost of care in the region (Swearingen, Schwartz, and Lee 1980).

The early emphasis of the program was on facility construction: Of the $49 million obligated through May 1970, $27 million had been devoted to construction (Swearingen, Schwartz, and Lee 1980). With time, the focus of the program broadened, and although construction continues to be important, the program now supports activities as diverse as medical residencies, sanitary landfills, and halfway houses for alcoholics. Currently, the majority of the funded projects strive to plan, initiate, coordinate, or systematize the delivery of primary-care services. Especially important have been programs to pioneer the use of mid-level health providers, such as nurse practitioners and physician assistants, and the development of systems to link primary care to secondary and tertiary sources of care (Kane, Dean, and Solomon 1978).

Rural-Health-Program Outcomes

There are two issues of primary relevance in regard to program outcomes: whether the programs are targeted to those populations identified as needy populations and whether they are achieving program goals.

The foregoing review of the methods by which programs are targeted and the description of program operations indicate that, in general, rural health programs are designed to respond to those populations defined as most in need. The Index of Medical Underservice, for example, takes into account infant mortality rates, percentages of elderly population (both groups have been identified as particularly vulnerable in the rural population), and poverty levels, as well as physician/population ratios, in the process of designating Medically Underserved Areas. The new Health-Manpower-Shortage Area (HMSA) designation criteria not only allow for the designation of facilities and institutions where concentrations of "at risk" persons may live (such as public institutions serving the elderly or federal prisons), but also, under some circumstances, have begun to take into account some within-area criteria such as infant mortality rates. Likewise, programs are designed under federal rural-health legislation specifically for two of the four "at risk" subpopulations which are generally agreed to have particular health needs, migrant workers and Appalachian people. Thus, it would seem, at least at a gross, national-policy level, that rural health programs are focused on those groups within the population most in need. Whether this holds true of particular communities where programs are located may be another matter.

The second question for program outcomes, then, is whether the rural health programs are achieving program goals. It has been difficult to demonstrate a direct relationship between rural health programs and access to care. The two national surveys by Aday and Anderson (1975) and Aday,

Anderson, and Fleming (1980) have shown improvements in access to care for virtually all groups within the United States population. But studies at the community level have found it difficult to link the increased availability of care under sponsored programs with measures of access (other than availability of providers). For example, a study by Hassinger and Hobbs (1972) of four Ozark communities with differing levels of available care found no significant differences in utilization of care among the communities. Hassinger and Hobbs (1972, p. 521) concluded that standards of care-seeking behavior existed in these rural communities which transcended the effect of supply:

> . . . among the communities a fairly uniform normative stance and common definition with regard to behavior associated with illness exists. As part of this definition, professional health services are regarded as legitimate and necessary in certain situations. On the basis of this normative-definitional stance, people will make considerable effort and utilize scarce resources in order to obtain medical services deemed needed in given situations.

These findings are consistent with the study by Luft, Hershey, and Morrell (1976) of the Livingston Community Health Services program in California, which found that health status, perceived health need, and a regular source of care were the primary determinants of utilization of care. Factors which were found to be unimportant were family income, price of services, and travel time to the source of care.

The recent study by Swearingen, Schwartz, and Lee (1980) for the Appalachian Regional Commission (ARC) concluded that ARC funding did increase the supply of physicians (measure of access) and that these communities did experience improvements in infant mortality rates (measure of health status). (The authors caution, however, that these conclusions are based on statistical correlations, which do not imply causation. That is, the increase in supply of physicians and the decrease in infant mortality could have occurred in these communities because of other reasons.) The study results still leave unanswered the issue raised by Hassinger and Hobbs of the link between supply of providers and utilization of services. That is, while it can be demonstrated that ARC funding increased the supply of physicians in the Appalachian region, there is no evidence that this can affect the health of Appalachian people unless they take advantage of the increased supply of physicians. Thus, if one is to assess the impact of these programs on the health of target populations, utilization is the key link. (It should be noted, however, that even when there is utilization, this may be an indication of improved access, but is no guarantee of improved health status.)

What, then, have been the experiences of rural health programs in regard to utilization by persons they are designed to serve? The results are not encouraging. Irrespective of the type of program sponsorship, few programs have become self-sufficient, few physicians are seeing patients at levels typical of national norms for all physicians or private rural physicians, and few programs experience high patient use by the communities they are designed to serve.

For example, the study for the ARC by Swearingen, Schwartz, and Lee (1980) found that of the twenty-one sites studied, only four were operating at or near capacity (ratio of actual visits to potential visits). The mean ratio for all the centers was 0.64—operating at slightly more than half capacity. Virtually all studies of government-supported rural health programs have recorded a low rate of patient use, a fact which is explored in this study, but which needs further exploration. Two means of highlighting utilization are discussed below—that of patient volume (practice use) and that of the proportion of persons in the community who come to the practice for care (penetration rate of the medical market).

Whether practice volume is measured in terms of physician productivity (number of encounters per hour or per year) or usage rates (number of visits per year to the practice that each patient makes), the message is clear that programs sponsored as part of the government's rural-health strategy have had difficulty encouraging patient use. This finding has been consistent since the very first evaluations of sponsored programs, and the evidence continues to mount.

One method of measuring use is physician productivity, usually defined as the rate of patients seen per hour or per year, or the number of patients seen compared to some national standard (the population taken care of by the physician), or the comparison of patients seen by private physicians and by those in government programs. On each of these measures, the conclusion is that physicians in government rural-health programs see few patients.

The Bureau of Community Health Services (BCHS) suggests that a full-time physician assignee have 4,200 office-based primary-care medical encounters per year (based on a 45-week year). This is considerably below the rate of patients seen by unsponsored primary-care physicians reported in several studies. In a 1973 survey of primary-care physicians, nonmetropolitan physicians saw an average of 8,443 patients annually, based on a 48-week year (American Medical Association, 1974). The American Medical Association (AMA) Center for Health Services Research and Development conducted a survey in 1972, dividing the providers by solo and two-physician practices. The solo physicians (metropolitan and nonmetropolitan combined) saw 6,085 patients annually, and those providers in two-physician practices saw 7,625 patients annually (AMA 1972).

One might argue that metropolitan physicians are always likely to have higher-volume practices, simply because of a larger population base from which to draw, and that it is inappropriate to average the volume of metropolitan and nonmetropolitan practices. Even if one accepts the 4,200 suggested standard of the BCHS as a national norm, however, most sponsored practices still have low practice volume. A study of West Virginia clinics with varying types of sponsorship (Holland et al. 1979) found only 44.2 percent saw patients at the government-suggested standard. Likewise, a study by the General Accounting Office (1978) of 110 NHSC sites found that physicians averaged 1.9 patients per hour, or about 3,000 visits per year for a 36-hour week at 44 weeks per year. Nighswander's (1977) sample of 80 NHSC sites (all had been in continuous operation for at least two years) found the average annual encounter rate to be 3,450.

When the patient volume of private-physician practices and that of government-sponsored rural practices are compared directly, the conclusion is the same: Sponsored physicians see far fewer patients. A 1975 study by Dobson et al. compared the use of forty-two private and NHSC practices in rural areas and found NHSC physicians saw only half as many patients per year as the private physicians (4,202 compared to 8,276). Approaching the comparison another way, Holland et al. derived a physician-capacity quotient from the literature on numbers of encounters per year typical of private primary-care physicians. Using 6,000 encounters per year as the chosen norm, Holland et al. conclude that the median value for percentage of physician capacity being used in the West Virginia sample was 65.5 percent.

Although studies of rural health programs have consistently reported the low practice use of sponsored programs, usually it has been researched as a part of studies of financial viability or self-sufficiency, rather than as a phenomenon in itself. This is because low utilization is a cause of subsequent low practice revenue and continued dependence on federal support. These studies yield inconclusive, and sometimes conflicting, explanations for the lack of self-sufficiency associated with low practice volume. A study of twenty NHSC practices in the Northwest by Rosenblatt and Moscovice (1978) identified four factors related to self-sufficiency of the practices and the ability to retain a physician: a service area with population over 4,000, the presence of a hospital, a group practice (at least two physicians) or peers, and completion of residency by the NHSC physician. Among the practices studied, the successful practices had service areas ranging from 6,800 to 9,600, whereas the practices with service-area populations under 4,000 stopped operating. Rosenblatt and Moscovice (1978, p. 760) suggest ". . . there is a minimum size service area below which physician practices cannot be expected to survive." Size of service area is closely related to two other important factors: presence of a group practice and existence of a hospital. All the practices that failed were solo practices in small towns without a hospital. The study's findings in regard to the residency training of physicians are more inconclusive, since four of the six practices which were able to convert to private practice had nonresidency-trained physicians, as did sixteen of the twenty practices where physicians left at the end of the two-year assignment (80 percent). Nevertheless, Rosenblatt and Moscovice feel this factor is an important one to consider in establishing new practices.

A study of sixty high and low utilizing practices by Nighswander (1977) concluded that a service area's sociodemographic characteristics were more important than the physician's personal characteristics or practice management and organization.[4] "Specifically, the age, educational level, wealth of the residents, and the density of the area are more important than physician attributes, community support, or the actual organization of the clinical setting" (Nighswander 1977, pp. 38-39). Nighswander reports that four variables explained 18 percent of the variation in patient visits per provider: percentage of the population greater than eighteen years of age, percentage of the population that was white, average family income, and county census. The only statistically significant variable was percentage of the population that was white. Nighswander offers no explanation for his findings except that they are similar to the detailed case study of Livingston, California, by Luft, Hershey, and Morrel (1976), who reported that low utilizers were differentiated from the high-utilization group by being poor and non-Anglo, having lower education, and being younger. The proximity of a hospital did not seem to make a difference, as it had in the Rosenblatt and Moscovice study. Of the sixty practices, there were equal numbers of low- and high-utilization practices in the groups defined as 1 to 9 miles from a hospital. Also of interest is the fact that two variables often suggested by the conventional wisdom of the rural health professionals—commitment of the physician to the community and level of community support—did not make a difference. Nighswander (1977, p. 40) concluded:

> The weight of evidence suggests that fixed community environmental characteristics are the most important factors associated with economic viability. These factors are ones that cannot be manipulated by the health care organization and might eventually result in the financial demise of a rural health care program.

A third study which examined self-sufficiency was that of Feldman, Deitz, and Brooks (1978). Again, this study was designed to test statistical associations between variables and the degree of self-sufficiency, and it offered few explanations for the results. Those variables significantly associated with self-sufficiency were control by a hospital, presence of laboratory tests (as measured by the dummy variable EKG), and prior level of self-sufficiency. Feldman, Deitz, and Brooks suggested that self-sufficiency is achieved by a "snow-balling effect" based, among other things, on levels of past self-sufficiency. But past self-sufficiency alone is not enough to explain current self-sufficiency, for if other variables do not contribute, it tends to level off at 0.75. This suggests that some practices would not achieve self-sufficiency even after many years and would continue to need outside support. Feldman, Deitz, and Brooks recommend that certain organizational changes be made to increase chances of self-sufficiency—hospital sponsorship, provision of laboratory tests as well as primary care, and public relations (which has a positive, but not statistically significant, effect).

Some of the variables exhibiting a negative impact were per capita income of the population (they posit that high-income people do not use government-sponsored clinics), which is a direct contrast to the Nighswander study; nonprofit status; and presence of outreach services which typically do not cover their costs.

Unlike the Nighswander study, which concluded that community variables were most important and organizational factors contributed little, if anything, to self-sufficiency, Feldman, Deitz, and Brooks stress the role of the funding agency in deciding if the practice is moving toward self-sufficiency and management changes, such as the provision of laboratory tests and hospital association, which can improve the statistical chances of self-sufficiency.

A final study which addressed issues of financial self-sufficiency and practice utilization is that of the General Accounting Office (GAO), which questioned the low utilization of NHSC physicians and recommended that DHEW change its methods of designating manpower-shortage areas. The low levels of use were attributed to the fact that the NHSC based its shortage designation primarily on a physician/population ratio of 1/4,000 (at that time) rather than ascertaining how many of the persons within the potential service area would utilize the new NHSC practice. The GAO report (1978, p. 36) concluded that low use was a result of lack of need in rural areas: "In our opinion, if the need for health manpower in these areas was truly critical, then one would expect NHSC physicians to be extremely busy or at least as busy as the average primary care physician in a non-shortage area."

The GAO report also recommended that inefficient utilization of staff and a low revenue/cost ratio be improved by not assigning more than one physician to a practice unless there were a demonstrated indication that two or more physicians would be utilized. This is a direct contrast to the Rosenblatt and Moscovice finding that the presence of two or more physicians was associated with self-sufficiency.

Although utilization levels have been identified as a key ingredient of self-sufficiency, another school of thought questions the revenue levels which can be generated from typical sponsored practices which emphasize office-based primary care. Several studies have suggested that the richness of the program inputs substantially affects revenue and income—and eventual self-sufficiency. The studies by Feldman, Deitz, and Brooks and by

Rosenblatt and Moscovice found that hospitalization was important to self-sufficiency. The Feldman, Deitz, and Brooks research also highlighted the importance of ancillary services. No research, however, has been able to systematically examine the range of program inputs across the total spectrum of sponsored programs and relate these to self-sufficiency. The study by Swearingen, Schwartz, and Lee (1980) for the ARC found that with the exception of hospital-based practices, few programs' physicians had hospital admitting privileges. This, however, may be unique to the states of Tennessee, West Virginia, and Pennsylvania, and not typical of all sponsored practices.

A final element in the self-sufficiency equation is program costs. There is some suggestion that the high costs of providing care in medically underserved areas could partially explain the difficulties rural sponsored practices have faced in becoming self-supporting. Two of the barriers to this analysis, however, have been the difficulty in obtaining reliable primary data relating to costs and the differing allocation of costs that have made study comparisons almost impossible. (This issue is discussed at greater length in chapter 4.) What is clear, however, is that costs are an important part of the options medical practices have in moving toward financial viability—improving revenues through greater practice volume or increased collections or reducing costs so that existing revenues are more adequate.

The Swearingen, Schwartz, and Lee study examined the relationships among cost, revenue, and collections. Of twenty-one practice sites examined, only one would have been self-supporting on patient-generated revenue alone. A major problem was low utilization—practice sites were operating at an average of 64 percent capacity. However, when practice revenues from 100 percent capacity were estimated, fourteen of the twenty-one centers would still operate at a loss, because costs per visit still exceeded revenue per visit at full capacity. (This assumes no change in fee schedules or collection policies or rates at full capacity.) Swearingen, Schwartz, and Lee attributed this dilemma to low revenues rather than excessive costs, however. They noted that charges were less than costs at all sites and that Medicare and Medicaid reimbursed for only a portion of true costs. [At the sites studied, Medicare and Medicaid reimbursement for a routine office visit did not exceed $6. The cost per visits for the center at capacity (all types of visits) ranged from $5.82 to $24.68.]

In another study, Dobson et al. (1975) examined these relationships and compared revenues and costs of NHSC practices during 1974 to data collected by the AMA on private physicians practicing in communities with population less than 50,000. Support costs for both types of physicians were nearly identical—approximately $34,000—suggesting to the researchers that there was little room for program efficiencies due to cost reduction.

Yet the NHSC cost per encounter was 58 percent higher than private physicians with young practices, because NHSC practice utilization was only half of the private utilization rate. If NHSC physicians had utilization rates comparable to those of private physicians, their cost per encounter would be approximately 30 percent lower than that of private physicians (because of a lower NHSC physician income, which reduces total practice costs). Dobston et al. suggested, however, that it is unlikely that NHSC physicians remaining in rural areas will have per encounter costs equal to those of private physicians if they maintain an NHSC style of practice which emphasizes high quality of care and moderate working hours.

A study by Heaton (1977) compared costs and revenues for 115 NHSC and 15 RHI sites. It found that NHSC practices were able to defray about 58 percent of their costs (including physician salaries) with revenues generated internally, while RHI sites were able to cover 52 percent of total costs. About 35 percent of the total sites examined covered less than 50 percent of their costs. Because of data limitations, the study was unable to develop a predictive model of demographic or site-specific variables by which to predict future practice performance. RHI sites had higher levels of productivity (attributed by the authors to more hours of patient contact) but had higher costs per encounter as well.

The evidence about the effect of cost on financial viability is less than conclusive—principally because typically practice volume has been so low that revenues covered only a small portion of costs. That is, some base-line costs are necessary for the operation of any medical practice. Even though direct and support costs of sponsored practices might not be excessive, revenues have been insufficient to cover these costs in a majority of cases. In addition, in the years since the major cost studies were completed by Heaton and Dobson, rural health policy has changed to encourage larger, more comprehensive programs that tend to include non-revenue-generating services, such as health education and outreach. Conclusions of existing research might be even less applicable to these current programs that have more substantial nonmedical costs.

What is clear from the foregoing discussion of rural-health-program outcomes is that very few definitive conclusions can be reached: it is difficult to demonstrate their effect on access (except if one defines improved access in terms of increased provider manpower, by definition an outcome of these programs). If one accepts the thesis that utilization is the key to understanding whether these programs affect access to care, one is hard pressed to find agreement on those factors which affect utilization of practices. The explanations of various authors range from community need, to management and organizational factors, to sociodemographic characteristics of the service area, to attributes of the providers.

Part of the problem in assessing the role of various factors in contributing to self-sufficiency may be that most studies have examined only sponsored practices. These are "biased" samples in the sense that revenue, utilization, and cost data for comparable self-sufficient practices are not available. Thus, even if one knows the utilization or cost levels for sponsored practices, there is no basis for comparison with practices which are similar, but self-supporting. The research design for this book attempts to correct this deficiency. The next chapter will discuss this methodology in some detail.

Notes

1. Primary medical-care manpower (including primary-care physicians, nurse practitioners, and physicians' assistants); dental manpower (including dentists and dental auxiliaries); psychiatric manpower (including psychiatrists and related practitioners providing mental health, alcohol, or drug-abuse services); vision-care manpower (including optometrists and ophthalmologists); podiatric manpower, pharmacy manpower; and veterinary manpower (with separate criteria for food-animal and companion-animal veterinarians) (Lee 1979).

2. For a complete description of the considerations, see Bureau of Health Manpower, "Report on Development of Criteria for Designation of Health Manpower Shortage Areas," Report No. 78-62, Hyattesville, Md., November 1977.

3. An exhaustive discussion of all public rural health programs is beyond the scope of this book. For example, the *Rural Health Clinic Services Act of 1977* (P.L. 95-210) is a financing mechanism rather than a program. Although its full impact has yet to be felt, it has the potential to make an important contribution to rural health care by amending the Social Security Act to allow for reimbursement (under certain circumstances) of mid-level health-care practitioners such as nurse practitioners and physician assistants under Medicare (Part B) and Medicaid. Likewise, the *Essential Community Facilities Loan Program* of the Farmers Home Administration makes low interest, 40-year loans available to towns of up to 10,000 population, and they may be requested for hospitals, clinics, and nursing homes as well as a number of other community facilities. These loans are often requested in connection with the other federal health programs discussed in the text. The *Health Maintenance Organization Program* was established under the Health Maintenance Organization Act of 1973 (P.L. 93-222) and provides grants, loans, and loan guarantees for feasibility, studies, planning, and initial HMO development. Although 20 percent of HMO funds are earmarked for nonmetropolitan areas, less than that is actually committed because few rural applicants qualify.

4. High utilizing sites were defined as those which had over 3,316 patient visits per year and which were not necessarily self-sufficient.

Study Design, Analytic Methods, and Practice Descriptions

Study-Design Rationale

The methodology for this research was designed to achieve several purposes: to examine in depth the components affecting practice self-sufficiency, to explore the effects of sponsorship on self-sufficiency, and to compare a limited number of practices on certain practice characteristics. The practices included were purposefully rather than randomly selected. This was done for the control of certain key variables which would yield information on specific research questions. A review of previous research conducted for this study (Carpenter and Gallagher 1978) concluded that a major problem was the use of secondary data, which had been submitted as part of government reporting requirements, or data compiled by the AMA for other purposes. Both sources proved unsatisfactory because the data are incomplete or inconsistent.[1] For example,

1. The lack of common definitions for such variables as encounters, cost centers, and so on makes comparisons across and among programs difficult, if not meaningless.
2. Study sites were often selected on the completeness of the reporting data, which could bias the sample, since it could be postulated that practices with better reporting systems are also better managed.
3. The reliance on already collected data limits the kind of questions researchers can ask because the importance of certain variables might not have been anticipated when the reporting system was designed, and the kinds of variables one needs to examine are different for management control than for research.
4. The lack of complete secondary data has caused at least two studies (Heaton, Rhodes, and Tindus 1976; Heaton 1977) to base their conclusions on data from a single fiscal quarter (since Heaton, Rhodes, and Tindus note an increase in morbidity and health-care utilization during the winter months, the annualized figures for this study are probably inflated).
5. Those studies (Dobson et al. 1975; Heaton, Rhodes, and Tindus 1976) which compared data from both publically sponsored and private providers had to perform numerous data adjustments since reported national data for private providers rarely conform to the categories or the specificity of breakdown used by government programs.

This literature review confirmed our opinion that at this stage in the state of the art, more would be learned from a limited number of in-depth practice visits in which primary data could be collected to answer certain research questions, than from a larger-scale survey with the same data limitations as previous inquiries. Purposeful practice selection thus became a key ingredient in the research.

By varying the practices studied according to size, geographic location, convenience of conducting a hospital practice, and the presence or absence of outside sponsorship, it was thought that wide differences in practice revenues, costs, and net income would emerge. The wide differences provide the opportunity to identify the significant factors of self-sufficiency.

The small number of practices included in the study, however, means that another sample of practices could yield somewhat different results and insights into the importance of the various factors. Therefore, including some safeguards that the findings did reflect the realities of rural-practice development was important. An advisory board composed of academics and practitioners was established and reviewed the process of nominating the practices to be studied.[2] The advisory board also reviewed the findings of the study as the site visit progressed. In addition, relevant and contemporary research findings were used as benchmarks whenever possible. It is important to understand, however, that no attempt has been made to generalize these findings to the experience of *all* rural practices. This research was exploratory—it attempted to examine variables and issues in a way impossible for previous research, but it does not comprise a statistically representative sample.[3]

A research limitation related to the use of secondary data is that the previously conducted analyses were confined to an examination of financial variables in isolation from other factors which affect viability. The research reported below utilized a more comprehensive approach:

1. Primary data collected from site visits to medical practices
2. Personal interviews with providers and support personnel
3. In-depth analyses of costs, revenues, patient encounters, and hospitalizations of each practice
4. Examination of the effects of practice-community relations, practice organization and management, and the scope and use of services offered on financial viability
5. Secondary, background data collected on demographic and economic characteristics of the practice service area

This more thorough data analysis provided an understanding of the current capacity of the practice, its history and development, and its relationship to other medical and nonmedical providers in the community.

One of the tradeoffs for the richness of data collected through in-depth site visits is the limited number of practices that can be studied and consequently the limited statistical interpretations that are appropriate. Throughout this book, practices are described in the very simplest statistical terms. In those instances where it was thought regression analysis or another statistical technique would be helpful in a research situation of larger numbers of practices, a methodological footnote has been added as an aid to future researchers.

Site Selection

The use of a limited number of in-depth practice analyses puts a premium on those practices selected for examination. Criteria guiding the site selection process were the following.

Different Practice Models

Two purposes of the research were to examine the components of self-sufficiency and to compare practice characteristics across a limited number of practices. Variations in the type of practitioner, including size of the practice and whether the practice made extensive use of hospital services, were assumed to be of critical importance in determining self-sufficiency. Models of practice organization selected for study were:

Solo-physician practice, hospital in town

Solo-physician practice, 20+ miles from a hospital

Group practice, hospital in town

Group practice, 10 miles from a hospital

Physician-extender practice

Matched Pairs of Practices

Why some practices were able to survive in rural areas on patient revenues alone while others needed ongoing support is another question explored by this book.

For five of the models, pairs of practices were selected which were matched as much as possible on sociodemographic characteristics of the service area; state, location, and maturity of practice; size of the service-area

population; and essential configuration of the practice. Table 2-1 outlines
the criteria met by each pair of practices. To permit examination of the effect of outside support on practice operations and thus on practice income,
each pair consisted of one practice receiving outside financial support
("sponsored practice") and the other existing on patient revenue alone
("unsponsored practice").

In order to examine a practice with a large Spanish-speaking population, it was decided to increase the number of practices to eleven. At the
same time, this provided the opportunity to examine a mini regional system
of one central practice and several full-time satellites, as well as a combination of the group-practice models, since the main practice was located in the
same town as a hospital, but the two satellite clinics shared a hospital
located a number of miles from each.[4] It was not possible to match this
practice to a nonsponsored practice having similar socioeconomic and
ethnic characteristics.

Since a prime consideration was to examine the components contributing to self-sufficiency, it was felt that the private practices (by definition already self-sufficient) should be matched with sponsored practices
that had a high likelihood of success. An elaborate process was developed to
identify practices which could become matched pairs and met all the other
research criteria, including geographic dispersion. As described below,
recommendations were obtained from a variety of knowledgeable sources
about practices which were perceived to be well located (high expectations
of self-sufficiency if not already self-sufficient) and relatively well managed
(stable, efficient providers of quality medical care). (Quality of care was not
a focus of the research. Knowledgeable sources were simply told to
nominate practices which, in their estimation, were providing good-quality
medical care.)

Because there was no source of readily available information which
could supply the level of detail necessary for such a specific site selection, a
nomination process was established with persons knowledgeable in the rural
health field. A minimum of three sources were contacted in each state where
practices were selected. An individual practice had to be independently
described and nominated by at least two sources to be considered for the
research. Information such as community demographics, which could be
verified from published data, was also obtained before the practices were
given final selection approval. The knowledgeable sources participating in
the site identification and nomination were staff from the Department of
Health, Education, and Welfare; the Appalachian Regional Commission;
the state health agencies; the state and local health systems agencies (HSAs);
the department of community medicine in medical schools within the state;
management consulting firms which provide technical assistance to rural
practices; state and local medical societies; and other academic researchers

who have surveyed medical practices; persons involved with organizations of rural health practitioners; and local physicians and hospital administrators.

Other Site-Selection Considerations

Previous research had already suggested that there are population levels below which practices cannot survive. In order to eliminate a lack of sufficient population as an explanation for practice nonviability, all the practices examined existed in service areas of more than the 4,000 population base suggested by Rosenblatt and Moscovice (1978).

Even in the most optimal situations, practice development requires that a practice be operating for some time at a level which creates credibility in the community. To control for the factor of practice immaturity as an explanation of low patient volume, we examined only practices with at least 1½ years of continuous history with the same provider. In addition, to attempt to eliminate a lack of management expertise as a possible explanation, the knowledgeable sources had been asked to nominate practices considered stable and well managed with high expectations for success.

A final issue related to the expected level of demand in the studied practices and the applicability of the findings to all rural areas. It is not within the scope of this book to become embroiled in the current debate which tries to draw distinctions between the demand for medical services in all rural areas and those which are governmentally classified as medically underserved. Chapter 3 summarizes the arguments over the measures used to designate medically underserved areas and health-manpower-shortage areas. Undoubtedly, researchers and practitioners will continue to make imprecise distinctions between the demand in all rural areas and those which can be considered "underserved" until some basic issues are resolved. For example, Wysong (1975) points out that when the University of Wisconsin was directed to develop the Index of Medical Underservice, the Department of Health, Education, and Welfare, the funding agency, had never defined what type of "underservice" the index was to measure. One might conceptualize underservice to mean areas where services are not available, or where they are not readily accessible, or where there is low use of available services, or where the outcome from using services is not acceptable.

Because we analyzed the self-sufficiency problems of practices which were often established by the federal government, all the practices either were officially designated by the federal government as being located in an HMSA or were matched on demographic, geographic, and socioeconomic characteristics to HMSAs. See table 4-1 for a description of this match of practices.

Table 4-1
Site Characteristics

Site	Service-Area Population	Demography by Service-Area Population[a] from 1970 Census				
		Percentage Black and Other Races	Percentage with Spanish Language Heritage	Persons Below Poverty Level	Location	Main Industry
Unsponsored group approximately 10 miles from hospital	One county	0.2	0.7	13.5	Northeast	Tourism, small college in town
Sponsored group approximately 10 miles from hospital	One county	0.3	1.8	11.0	Northeast	Tourism, small college in town
Unsponsored group with hospital in town	One county	5.6	1.1	13.2	West	Logging and wood production, manufacturing
Sponsored group with hospital in town	One county	0.7	0	8.4	West	Logging
Sponsored solo 20+ miles from hospital	Two counties	0.2 0.1	0.5 0.3	12.8 7.7	Midwest	Family farms, small seed company
Unsponsored solo 20+ miles from hospital	Three counties	1.5 0.1 0.1	0.3 0.2 0.6	10.8 14.0 11.1	Midwest	Family farms
Unsponsored solo with hospital in town	One county	32.2	0	40.8	South	Agriculture, pulp mill
Sponsored solo with hospital in town	One county	31.4	0	35.8	South	Agriculture
Sponsored group with two satellite clinics, hospital in town	Three counties	1.6 0.7 1.1	33.7[b] 67.6[b] 78.5[a]	21.5 42.0 36.0	Southwest	Agriculture, some tourism

Sponsored physician-extender clinic	Two counties	26.1	1.2	22.0	Mid-Atlantic	Agriculture, some textile industry, some wood-products manufacturing
		34.8	0.2	35.2		
Unsponsored physician-extender clinic	Four counties	43.4	0	44.8	Mid-Atlantic	Agriculture, some pulp and paper, some fishing, some tourism
		7.3	0.4	16.4		
		41.5	0.1	29.2		
		12.5	4.6	13.7		
Total United States		12.5	4.6	13.7		
Total Non-metropolitan		10.4	2.6[b]	19.2		

[a] The service areas of some sites contained parts of more than one county. In those cases, the demography of each county involved is presented.
[b] Includes persons of Spanish language plus persons of Spanish surnames not speaking Spanish.

Instruments for Data Collection

Three instruments were developed to collect data. A *community profile* for demographic, community, and medical trade-pattern data was completed prior to a site visit. The data were obtained from the Census Bureau, state and local health planning agencies, local medical societies, and the specific clinics' grant applications. The community profile was designed to double-check how accurately each pair of sites was matched, to discover any special health needs or characteristics in a site's service area, and to collect demographic and socioeconomic status data for later analysis.

Interview guides were used by the research team to conduct on-site interviews with physicians, physician extenders, administrators, and advisory board members. The guide was designed to explore community-practice relations, practice organization, history and "mission," and practice management.

The *practice profile* assembled data describing the actual operations of each practice. One section of the profile asked questions about numbers and kinds of employees, size of facilities, services offered, and other organizational information—to be answered by a physician, an administrator, or a bookkeeper at each site. The remaining part of the profile collected detailed, specific information about charges per revenue center, collections per revenue center, cost per revenue center, use of each revenue center, and total practice use. For these categories, data were collected on site for later compilation. As a rule, data collected at the practice had to be reassembled to provide the uniform categories asked for on the profile.

Collection of Raw Data

We compiled raw data concerning charges, payments, and service procedures from one of three systems typically used by individual practices. At those practices where a one-write pegboard-sheet system was used to tally services, four months out of each year studied were sampled—February, May, August, and November. (This is a system by which pressure-sensitive paper provides a statement to the patient, a record for the practice, and an entry for the daily log sheet in one writing operation.) Data were collected for each service center studied; they served as a basis by which "actual" accounting information could be apportioned to these centers. At those practices which used a computerized system, data were collected for the entire year. Some computer systems summarized data in categories not usable for our research. In other practices, data concerning charges, payments, and service procedures were compiled by an individual who played a significant role in the management of the practice, usually an administrator, a bookkeeper, or an accountant.

Practice use, charge, and collection data used in this book were computed from the charge, payment, and service-procedure data compiled on site. Information concerning practice use, practice growth in terms of numbers of patients, and patient coverage by third-party reimbursement sources was extracted directly from a survey sample of each practice's patient files. The sample size was 5 percent.

Every effort practicable was made to obtain accurate data from each practice. An audit was *not* performed, however, and the accuracy of the data was dependent on the record-keeping and accounting methods of each practice.[5] The integrity of the data was also dependent on uniform definitions of terms such as *encounter* among practices. For those practices where data were obtained directly from daily log sheets, common definitions could be easily maintained. For those practices using other types of data-collection methods, we ascertained whether there were any important definitional differences that would prevent data being compared. Explanatory notes, where appropriate, are provided in the tables.

Financial-Data Analysis

A number of assumptions had to be made in regard to the financial data of the eleven practices: the basis on which each practice's financial data were evaluated, the use of collections to approximate realizable revenues, the assumed behavior and categorization of costs, and the accrual and allocation of costs.

It was necessary to develop a common base on which the financial data of the eleven practices could be evaluated. For example, some of these practices accounted for themselves as corporations, others as nonprofit organizations, and still others on a sole proprietorship/partnership basis. To present data in a comparable format, the financial data for each practice were stated in terms of a sole proprietorship/partnership model, which enabled comparisons of each practice relative to the income it was able to generate for the physician(s).

Collections were used as a basis of revenue measurement for a variety of reasons. Normally, charges adjusted for losses due to bad debts and third-party reimbursement would be used as revenues. However, most practices did not accurately account for these losses, and the use of charges without adjustment would have resulted in an overstatement of practice income. Other reasons for using collections to measure revenues include (1) the assumption that collections should approximate realizable charges over a fiscal year, (2) the inability to accurately evaluate the realizable value of the accounts receivable and related losses for each practice, and (3) the common accounting practice among physician practices of using the cash basis in recording revenues and expenses.

To determine a relative value of each service category to the practices, a "contribution" was calculated for each category wherever possible. This contribution allows the user to see the relative profitability of each category in terms of the net benefit produced to the practice. This benefit or contribution is measured as simply the revenue less the variable costs associated with each category.

In deriving this contribution, all medical and administrative expenses were considered variable and matched to each category. Medical materials and fees were matched directly to each category. Nonphysician medical labor was apportioned to these categories based on the estimated amount of time these people spent in each category. Administrative costs were apportioned on the basis of the number of times care was given to patients in each category. While the above methods of allocation are somewhat imprecise, they serve as a consistent basis of comparison and do provide an approximation of the amount of contribution per category.

Limitations of the Data

Limitations of the data are of two types. First, as discussed above, the decision to conduct intensive practice analyses enhances the richness of the data, but reduces the number of practices studied. Our findings are based on only eleven medical practices. Second, research findings are sensitive to the assumptions made in compiling the data. For example, because accounting methods used by the practices were not uniform, standard cost categories were developed and practice costs were assigned to these categories.

It was assumed that collections more closely approximate realizable revenues than unadjusted charges. Typically, collections underestimate realizable revenues while gross charges overstate this amount; however, the use of collections results in a closer approximation and a more conservative (theoretically preferable) approach.

Total collections were allocated to the various revenue categories on the basis of the sampling done at each practice. This assumes a uniform collection rate among the service categories of each practice.

Cost data were taken directly from the income statements prepared by each practice. In many cases, further investigation was necessary to obtain a breakdown of certain costs into the categories studied. An assumption that had to be made was that cash-based records would approximate theoretically preferred, accrual-based records for those practices where the cash basis was used. This assumes equivalent amounts of inventory at the beginning and the end of the fiscal year, and the validity of the cost data for most of the practices rests on this assumption.

Costs were categorized as medical, administrative, and plant. Medical costs are those which were directly related to servicing patients. These included all direct materials, fees, and medical labor (other than that of the physician). Administrative costs were all indirect, variable costs incurred by the practices, in essence, all costs that were neither plant nor directly related to medical care. Plant costs include items such as insurance, facilities, utilities, accounting, legal, and equipment expenses.

Practice Descriptions

An important element of this research is the in-depth analysis of matched pairs of practices, each pair representing a model of medical-care delivery and meeting certain criteria for research. This section presents a brief description of the practices visited.

Group Practice 10 Miles from a Hospital

Both practices representing this model are located in New England towns of population less than 2,000, with tourism, light industry, and agriculture as the main industries. A small liberal arts college located in the town is an important source of patients for each practice. The service area for both practices is about 10,000 population, almost exclusively white, with poverty levels of 11 and 13 percent. The attending physicians for both practices are male in their mid to late thirties, with training in general and/or internal medicine. In both practices, the providers had chosen their particular practices over other options.

The *unsponsored practice* began in 1973 as a National Health Service Corps site (designation for NHSC eligibility initiated by the physicians) and converted to private practice in 1975. A second physician, a native of the town, had joined the practice in 1974, and a third (not included in the data) had come in 1977. The physicians provide backup to a nurse practitioner housed on the college campus. The only other practitioner in the service area had retired about a year after the practice had converted from NHSC status. The physicians own the office facility, a recently renovated Victorian house (with separate office space rented to a psychologist and a rental apartment in the rear of the house) on a main street of the town. The town is a small trading center for the area, with markets, a pharmacy, a bank, and some retail shops. The practice location is in the southern third of its geographic area, with the admitting hospital outside the service area 10 miles farther south in a town of about 8,500. It is a modern 100 + bed facility. This practice has been self-supporting since 1974. The main contribution to profitability (approximately 38 percent) is hospital revenues. Partly because of moderate practice costs, revenues have been more than sufficient to support two physicians. Net income per physician has fallen with the addition of the third physician. The main reason for adding another provider was increased personal time.

The *sponsored practice* is an outgrowth of the local college's desire to expand its campus medical facilities to a community-based program after being unable to retain campus physicians. In 1973 a physician was recruited to both provide medical care at the college and conduct a part-time community feasibility study. In 1974 the program began operation on a small scale in a college building, with CETA workers as support personnel. In 1975 a grant was received from the regional medical program, and a second physician and a physician assistant were added as well as an administrator. In 1976 foundation funding began which solidified the clinician-administrator model. A community board had been elected in 1975 which began plans for a new facility financed by locally raised and foundation monies. This building, which also provides space for a psychologist intern, a dentist, a health educator, a pharmacy, and community meetings, was opened in September 1978. It is adjacent to the college campus on the outskirts of town. The town is not a retail trade center, but rather a passing-through point on a main road linking a larger town with other parts of the state. A post office is the only major facility near the practice, although there is the possibility of other facilities in the future. There are no other providers in the service area, although several physicians live in the area and practice in the nearby large town of 19,000, where the hospital is located. The practice is located in the southwestern third of the service area, with the admitting hospital another 10 miles to the west. It is a modern, 185-bed facility.

This practice is an example of the administrator model, which has generated high administrative costs but also substantial income through grant support. The providers' personal philosophy of medical-care delivery deemphasizes hospital care. The combination of high administrative costs and lack of hospital revenue existing simultaneously with a low office-visit rate per physician ensures the need for continuing grant support. During the course of our research, the physicians applied to the NHSC. For the sake of comparability with other practices, auxiliary services (dental, pharmacy, psychological counseling) were not included in revenues or encounters. Medical and administrative costs associated with these categories also were excluded. (This was done by a staff estimate of the amount of personnel time devoted to these categories as well as to produce cost records.)

Solo Physicians Located More than 20 Miles from
a Hospital

Both practices representing this model are located in towns of population less than 2,000 in a farming area of the Midwest known for the richness of the soil and the stability of the farming population. Family farms are the predominant industry, with grain and seed companies and service occupations providing some jobs. Both practices serve populations of approximately 5,000 to 6,000 and are located in more than one county. All the concerned counties have minority populations of less than 2 percent.

The *sponsored practice* was formed as a result of a community effort to recruit a dentist. A young osteopath finishing his residency and about to begin his NHSC obligation was interested in the community because he had relatives in the area and had also gone to college in the nearby large city. At the initiation of the interested physician, the community was certified as an eligible NHSC placement. The community had also been trying to recruit a physician through private channels for several years. The NHSC physician entered practice in 1977, assuming the facilities and hiring the receptionist of a retiring physician who had been in practice in the community for forty years. The service area of approximately 6,000 people cuts across three counties. Although there are no other practitioners within the service area, there are several providers in other parts of each of the counties. Both the existing office space and a new medical center/community center being built by the community are on the main street of the town, a small trade center for the county. The community is considered to be a progressive one, with several retail stores, a library, a bank, a pharmacy, churches, a seed company, and a grain elevator.

Because of the distance from the city where the hospital is located (23 miles) the physician does not have a hospital practice, but refers to specialists in the hospital city. It is a 320-bed facility located in a metropolitan area with a population of 113,000. There are also two other hospitals within approximately the same distance where the physician could hospitalize. A hospital practice was to be started shortly with the arrival of a surgeon who is fulfilling his military obligation. This practice had a net income in excess of $20,000 from operations in its first full calendar year. Since the physician was not billing for the full cost of ancillary services, the net income would probably have been higher if the physician were private.[6] Also, hospital revenues now lost through referrals would be retained by the practice once a second physician were added.

The *unsponsored practice* is the result of the community's effort to recruit a physician since the last provider's departure in 1972. In 1977, they were successful in attracting an osteopath just finishing his residency in the state who had decided he wanted to practice in a rural area. The community committee was influential in arranging for office space on the main street of the town, next to the bank, and for loans for office equipment and a house. As a result of the physician's presence, a pharmacy opened in the town, which was not otherwise a trade center for the county. The main industry in town is a farm-implement dealership that has a large dollar volume but does not attract large numbers of customers.

During the intervening years when there had been no provider in town, the people in the service area of approximately 5,000 persons patronized physicians in the larger hospital towns up to 25 miles away. Getting persons to change their medical behavior proved more difficult than anticipated. When the volume of the practice did not meet expectations, the physician opened a part-time office in a nearby small town, in a medically equipped trailer provided by a local family. He also identified home deliveries of children as an unmet need in the service area and provided this as a special service. The practice is located 21 miles from the 222-bed hospital in a city of 31,000 where the physician conducts his hospital practice. Because of the distance from the hospital, the physician had developed a moderate emergency facility in his own office. During the time the physician is at the satellite clinic or making hospital rounds, his wife, a nurse, covers the office for him. Even with these efforts and some public support by local leaders, the physician was unable to develop a financially viable practice because of low patient volume. After 3 years in the community, he left to begin a new practice closer to a hospital.

Low volume (less than 4,000 total encounters per year) was the factor inhibiting financial self-sufficiency. The other criteria to be discussed as leading to self-sufficiency—high proportion of hospitalization, high average price per encounter, high collection rate, good cost management—were exhibited by this practice.

Group Practices with Hospital in Town

Both practices representing this model are located in towns of the Rocky Mountain West with population less than 2,000. Lumbering and wood products are the major industries. Both practices serve a geographic area of one county defined primarily by the mountain ranges. The service-area population is almost exclusively white, despite the nearby presence of a large Indian reservation. The unsponsored practice serves a somewhat larger county (8,000) that is poorer (13 percent) and has a larger Indian population (5 percent) than the sponsored practice with 4,000 population, 8 percent poverty rate, and less than 1 percent Indian population. The sponsored practice also serves a significant transient population from an interstate highway, a major East-West trucking and travel route. Both practices are located in towns which serve as small trade centers with retail stores, banks, pharmacies, and food markets, although only one practice is located in the county seat. Both practices have all-weather access to a metropolitan area of 65,000 with three hospitals and numerous specialists. This referral center is located 75 miles away for the unsponsored practice and 50 miles away for the sponsored. The attending physicians for both practices are male, with the physicians in the unsponsored practice somewhat older than those of the sponsored practice.

The *unsponsored practice* began in 1968 when two local families donated $50,000 and land to establish a clinic. Within the first year, a part-time office was opened in another small town (the county seat) at the urging of the community. The practice continues to staff this office on a rotating basis, although there is some feeling on the part of administrative staff that this is being done more for improved access to care than for the additional business generated by this office. In 1970 a private proprietary hospital was built in the practice town (containing twenty beds and a ten-bed nursing home unit) to replace a Hill-Burton hospital elsewhere in the county that the county government was unable to support. The practice physicians were instrumental in generating community support for the hospital, and they have some financial interest in it. The nursing-home section of the hospital is now being enlarged. The original physicians were a general surgeon and an internist who had developed surgical skills. When the surgeon left in 1975 to move to a larger city, he was replaced by another physician with surgical skills, an internist who had left a large city practice after seventeen years and then had an unsuccessful start as a solo physician in another small town. A third physician, an orthopedist, was added in 1977; he was to provide orthopedic backup to physicians on the Indian reservation one day per week. There are no other physicians in the service area. The office facility is an enlarged version of the original clinic building, located in a residential area several blocks from the center of town. The hospital is located on the outskirts of town. The practice town is in the eastern third of the county-wide service area.

This practice has the highest net income per physician of any practice studied. This was due primarily to a high proportion of hospitalization, capacity for surgery, and a low proportion of referrals outside the service area. Patient volume was sufficient to generate high physician income, despite substantial administrative costs.

The *sponsored practice* is an outgrowth of a medical practice with a somewhat erratic history that had existed in the county seat for some years. In 1969 the resident physician convinced the county government to pass a bond issue to build a new hospital because the old one was in violation of health and safety regulations. These plans were abandoned, however, when the physician was injured in an automobile accident and discontinued practice. A new physician recruited in 1971 left in 1972 for personal reasons. A foreign medical graduate from Greece also practiced in the town temporarily, but did not stay. Medical services were provided by a series of visiting physicians until 1974 when the first NHSC physician arrived. The county arranged for clinic services to be provided from a medically equipped trailer located next to the hospital. The threat of the physician to leave if a new hospital was not built stimulated the county to plan for a new hospital. (The hospital is a ten-bed facility with a twenty-bed nursing-home unit.) A hospital-management firm which had managed the new hospital since its opening also took over management of the clinic in 1977. The original NHSC physician remains with the practice, beginning his fourth year of service at the time of the practice visit. The second physician assigned left within a few months for personal reasons. A third NHSC physician fulfilled his commitment and then left for private practice in an adjoining state. A fourth physician, who arrived in July 1978, plans to leave after his NHSC assignment to complete residency training. In order to use all the available facilities of the hospital, an orthopedist had been contracted from the near-by large city to provide specialty care and do surgery one day per week, beginning the week of the practice visit. To increase the size of the practice to a three-physician group, this physician was expected to arrive within a few weeks after the practice visit and thus is not included in the data. The hospital board had also recruited a private physician with three years of surgical training. The hospital is located at the edge of town. The practice is centrally located in the countywide service area.

This practice requires continuing grant support. Low patient volume (sufficient at this point to support one physician) generates a moderate proportion of hospitalization, but the absence of surgery and of sophisticated in-patient care limits the revenue per hospital encounter. All ancillary services are performed in the hospital, depriving the practice of this source of revenue. Costs are relatively moderate, despite somewhat high administrative costs.

Solo Physician with Hospital in Town

Both practices representing this model are located in the Deep South in towns of 2,000 to 3,000 with significant black (31 to 32 percent) and poverty (35 to 40 percent) populations. Agriculture is the main industry in both one-county service areas of 10,000 to 11,000. A pulp mill also provides some employment in the county of the unsponsored practice. The physicians for both practices are male, in their mid to late thirties, with training in family and general medicine. Both specifically chose to locate in their respective communities.

The *unsponsored practice* began in 1977 as a result of a recruitment effort by leaders in the county seat (population 2,200) to improve services in the county hospital and give relief to one physician with a full practice (on the recruitment committee) and another who was cutting back his practice because of age. A young family practitioner had returned to his hometown 20 miles away and was working on a salaried basis with an established physician. He was interested in moving to a smaller community where he could have his own practice. A contract with the county guaranteed his salary for one year, assisted with the rent on a fully equipped clinic facility as well as located a home for him. The practice was self-sufficient, since a modest salary was guaranteed within the first year. The county seat is centrally located in the county, about 20 miles from a larger community of 11,000 with a hospital and several specialists. A metropolitan area of 150,000 with several hospitals and a medical school is 60 miles away. The hospital used by the physician is a relatively modern, 47-bed facility currently undergoing some renovation and expansion. The three physicians in the town share calls. The office facilities consist of a modern, one-story clinic built by the previous physician in a residential section of town. The physician's wife is a nurse who assisted in the establishment of the practice and still works there part-time on a nonsalaried basis.

This practice exhibits all the qualities found necessary for self-sufficiency, except for a relatively low collection rate. High practice volume plus good cost management, coupled with a high proportion of hospitalization, yielded a net practice income in excess of $40,000.

The *sponsored practice* is a component of a larger community-development effort by a religious group which has had missionary activities in the state since 1960, primarily aimed at improvements within the black community.

The health program and a number of other community-development ventures are located in the county seat (population 2,800) of a one-county service area of approximately 10,000. Health-related activities (physicians and health screening) which had been done on a sporadic basis since 1969 became a regular service in 1975 when a physician (a pediatrician) arrived for a full-time, two-year missionary assignment. Later in the year, the program moved from temporary clinic facilities in the black section of town to a purchased clinic building in the heart of town across the street from the county courthouse—viewed as an important symbol that the program was attempting to serve all the people of the service area. In 1976 an NHSC physician joined the program. He had learned of the church's missionary work while doing his residency and had been instrumental in having the program designated as NHSC-eligible. He intends to remain in the community permanently. The other provider at the site is a pediatric nurse practitioner who had come as an RN in 1973 and had gone through RNP training in the state in 1975. She has assumed a greater role in pediatric care since the departure of the pediatrician in 1977. There are four other physicians in the town. Two are semiretired with limited practices of 25 to 50 percent. One is a full-time general practitioner. The fourth is a newly placed NHSC physician, a surgeon assigned to the private general practitioner. Calls at the local hospital are shared among the three full-time physicians. The hospital is a Hill-Burton structure with fifty-bed capacity. The practice is located 25 miles from a metropolitan area (population 150,000) with several referral hospitals and a medical school.

The non-self-sufficiency of this practice is due in part to a low revenue per encounter ($8.04)—a composite of low charge per encounter ($10.90) plus a low collection rate (73.7 percent). Costs seem to be high in all categories. Part are unreimbursed outreach costs of $14,000. Administrative costs were high despite services contributed without charge from the administrator of a regional Rural Health Initiative (RHI) grant. Patient volume was not sufficient to support both a physician and a nurse practitioner.

Sponsored Group Practice with Satellite Clinics in a Spanish-Speaking Population

This practice serves a large, sparsely populated, three-county area with a total population of about 26,000. The percentage of Spanish-speaking or -surnamed persons in these counties ranges from 33 to 78 percent. The proportion of the population living in poverty is also high, from 21 to 42 percent. Agriculture is the main industry, with tourism also providing some jobs.

The main clinic and the two satellites have had quite different histories. The counties with the satellites are very sparsely populated and poor. They have had some type of sponsored medical services since the 1960s. The main practice assumed operation of clinic A in 1976 and clinic B in 1977. The main practice was organized in 1976 as the medical component of a rural health maintenance organization (HMO). This had been developed partly as a response to the fact that existing medical practices in the community of 7,000 were full and partly as a result of the desire of some private physicians to link services between this larger community and the very rural outlying areas. When the HMO converted to an Independent Practice Association (IPA) model, however, the need for a district medical component for the HMO was eliminated. The practice now operates under contract to the HMO, as well as accepts non-HMO patients. All the medical staff are NHSC employees, some obligated and others civil servants. The practice also has RHI and other health grants. The initial physician was joined by a second physician and three nurse practitioners in 1976. By the end of 1977, the initial physician and two of the nurse practitioners had left, to be replaced by two physicians (one a Chicano native to one of the satellite towns). A fourth physician arrived in 1978 for a total of four physicians and one nurse practitioner serving the three clinics. All the providers live in the large town of the main practice and staff the satellite clinics on a rotating basis. There is also a full-time administrator for the practice. The services for all three sites are centrally administered, with uniform purchasing and billing procedures.

The main practice operates in a town of 7,000, which is a major trade center for the area with retail shops, banks, other small businesses, and a junior college as principal employers. The clinic offices are in a modern, one-story facility centrally located in the town. The hospital used by the practice is a modern, seventy-bed facility. Clinic A is located 30 miles to the south of the main practice in a town of 1,100. The clinic, which is on the outskirts of town, had its origins in the Office of Economic Opportunity (OEO) health-centers program and has been operated and staffed by the main practice since 1976. Clinic B, located 60 miles to the southeast of the main practice, uses part of a very large facility which was also part of the OEO health-centers program. It is situated by itself, outside town. The hospital used by the two satellite clinics is located halfway between the two towns. It is an older, forty-three-bed facility. There are also two other small, older hospitals of forty- and fifty-seven-bed capacities in the service area, both operating at 30 to 40 percent occupancy rate. The referral hospital used by the practice is located 90 miles away in a city of over 100,000. It is a multispecialty hospital. This practice is an example of the regional-administrator model, with one administrator who makes basic personnel and other administrative decisions for the entire practice.

The revenues of the central practice and two satellite clinics suffer from insufficient patient volume, low collection rates, and relatively high costs. Especially prominent is the amount paid for nonphysician medical labor and the amount for administrative salaries.

Physician-Extender Practices

Both practices representing this model are located in coastal mid-Atlantic states with forestry, manufacturing (predominantly textiles), and agriculture as the major industries. There are large minority populations in each multicounty service area (7 to 43 percent), and the number of persons living in poverty is also quite large (16 to 44 percent). For both practices, the use of a physician extender is a model of medical care new to the community. Both providers (one a physician assistant and the other a family nurse practitioner) are male and in their middle thirties. The supervising physicians, located in larger towns 20 and 30 miles away, are all male and in their middle to late thirties.

The *sponsored practice* is the result of community efforts by a town of less than 1,000 that had been unable to recruit a physician. The town leaders had been in negotiation with several nearby communities to see if they could jointly recruit a physician, but in 1975 decided to apply for a program through a state agency by which they could receive developmental funding for a primary-care clinic to be staffed by a physician extender. The new clinic building, which has been built on the outskirts of town, is the result of an extensive community fund-raising effort to meet the local-match requirements. At the same time, the state agency also provided scholarship opportunities for trained medical personnel to become physician extenders through local universities. A resident of a nearby community who had had military medic training had returned to the state and finished nursing school. He had graduated from the family-nurse-practitioner training at the time the clinic was ready to begin operation. The third component of the program is the supervising physician practice, which was arranged through the state agency. It is composed of three young physicians who had been stationed in the area while fulfilling military obligations and who decided to establish a group practice. Their practice opened shortly before the clinic began operation. Their supervision of the nurse practitioner was daily at first and has since been reduced to one-half day per week. At the time of the site visit, the supervising practice was still receiving a retainer from the extender site for their services. Most referrals for hospitalization are made to the supervising practice, although this is not a condition of the relationship.

This practice suffers from inadequate patient volume. It exhibits all the other criteria for financial success found in the self-sufficient practices (good cost management, high collection ratio, and adequate revenue per encounter). Laboratory tests are a profit center for this practice, a condition not found in any of the self-sufficient practices. Lack of revenue from hospitalized patients and low patient volume account for the deficit of $17,000 per year.

The *unsponsored practice* is a component of a physician practice in another town, about 30 miles away, with several more physician-extender clinics planned as part of an expansion program to take place under federal support. Unlike the other practices discussed, therefore, it will move from unsponsored self-sufficiency to a sponsored relationship in the future. The extender practice has been in existence since 1976 when two physician assistants were recruited by a local physician who had been in the community for eleven years. By the time the two physician assistants had arrived in May 1976, however, the physician had left and the practice was taken over by a radiologist until September 1977. During this time the patient load decreased sharply, partly because the radiologist was not able to develop a primary-care practice. When that physician left in September 1977, the 35-bed hospital closed. The present supervising physician made a proposal to the community recommending that the extender practice be operated in the clinic facilities of the closed hospital. The practice reopened in January 1978. The difficulties in rebuilding patient volume are attributed to the break in service and the fact that many of the patients were chronic-care patients who needed to find other providers immediately. During this same transition, the supervising physician visited the practice one day per week. Patients were referred to the supervising practice for hospitalization in the larger town or for more extensive laboratory work.

This practice encountered numerous problems in compiling accounting data during the fiscal year. Accounting entities used were different from those examined by us. General trends of practice operation were discernible, but limits must be drawn on the specificity of conclusions. This practice was especially laboratory-intensive. Laboratory revenue accounted for 23 percent of total revenues. Laboratories are a profit—33 percent of revenues from laboratories are practice income. This physician-extender practice, as a separate entity, expected to be near the break-even point in the near future.

Notes

1. For a more complete discussion of these problems, see Carpenter and Gallagher 1978.

2. The members of this advisory board are listed in the Acknowledgments to the book.

3. It should be noted that no research up to this time had been statistically representative. The first data universe from which a representative sample could be drawn was compiled in 1979 and published in February 1980 under the title *Directory of Rural Health Care Programs* (DHEW, Office of the Assistant Secretary for Planning and Evaluation/Health). This is part of a larger study of funded programs, the National Evaluation of Primary Health Care Programs, conducted by the Health Services Research Center, University of North Carolina.

4. It should be noted that several of the other practices have office hours available in another town, usually on a very part-time basis. These were not considered to be regional systems. Except when noted, they are treated as a single practice.

5. Accounting data were cross-referenced with audited financial statements, tax returns, and reports filed with other government agencies, where possible. No further verification was attempted. Accounting methods were not the same for each practice, and the validity of the data depends on the competence and integrity of the accounting and administrative personnel of each practice as well as the research team's understanding and interpretation of their methods.

6. The physician had taken over a traditional-style practice where almost no ancillary services had been performed for many years. He realized that his prices did not cover costs, but felt that prices had to remain modest to introduce the service to the community. He expressed the opinion that if he were a private physician, he would have to raise ancillary prices to cover costs.

Research Findings on Financial Self-Sufficiency and Sponsorship

Continuing debate centers on the choice of the most appropriate long-range goal for federally sponsored rural health practices, self-sufficiency or efficiency. Self-sufficiency, the original programmatic goal, has been supplanted by efficiency for publicly sponsored practices, as policymakers have witnessed the myriad of difficulties inherent in rural-practice development. Self-sufficiency stresses the "bottom line," that is, net practice income or income available to the physician. Efficiency emphasizes productivity and low administrative costs. If health needs are being met though delivered in the least expensive manner, but revenues remain inadequate, a strong case can be made for continued special assistance. The inadequate revenue might result from inadequate volume because of the sparcity of the population or because the type of medical services provided is not adequately reimbursed.

This chapter describes the practices studied according to their self-sufficiency status. The next chapter highlights the differences in efficiency of sponsored and unsponsored practices. Significant overlap exists in the data discussions since only one of the non-self-sufficient practices is unsponsored. Nevertheless, distinct discussions are merited given the public-policy interests in self-sufficiency and efficiency.

Practice Self-Sufficiency

Self-sufficiency remains a focus of health policy. The growth of a newly established rural practice to self-sufficiency status will allow government and other sponsors to extricate themselves from having to financially guarantee the viability of these practices ad infinitum. Self-sufficiency may become even more important as limited government and private resources must be allocated among a growing array of providers and programs.

This analysis of eleven rural medical practices has yielded an extraordinarily wide range of variation on the dimension of degree of practice self-sufficiency. Table 5-1 illustrates this range, ranking these practices on the basis of net practice income available per physician. The net-practice-income figures do not include grant or other subsidy support, and therefore, they reflect what would be available for physician salaries before these special awards. In the case of sponsored practices, which often had large negative net incomes, physicians had guaranteed salaries between

Table 5-1
Rank of Practices by Degree of Self-Sufficiency plus Other Related Measures

Rank	Practice	Net Practice Income per Physician[b]	Total Revenues per Physician[b]	Total Costs per Physician[b]	Office Encounters per Physician	Total Encounters per Physician	Average Price per Encounter
1	Unsponsored group, hospital in town	$60,263	$121,358	$61,095	4,901	7,919	$18.55
2	Unsponsored group, 10 miles from hospital	36,613	76,960	40,347	5,158	6,971	11.98
3	Unsponsored solo physician, hospital in town	33,530	97,607	64,077	5,193	7,581	15.66
4	Sponsored solo physician, 20+ miles from hospital	20,415	93,319	72,904	7,530	7,620	13.44
5	Sponsored group, hospital in town	9,929	50,707	40,778	3,454[c]	4,231	14.10
6	Unsponsored solo physician, 20+ miles from hospital	6,715	57,942	51,227	3,207	3,814	16.19
7	Sponsored extender practice[a]	(17,420)	39,800	57,220	3,510	3,510	12.11
8	Unsponsored extender practice[a]	(19,086)	86,507	105,593	NA[d]	NA	NA
9	Sponsored group, 10 miles from hospital	(35,490)	53,408	88,898	3,966	4,162	15.05
10	Sponsored group with two satellite clinics	(38,145)	54,811	92,956	4,248	4,990	14.76
11	Sponsored solo physician, hospital in town	(64,446)	57,520	121,966	5,469	7,158	10.90
	Average of all practices studied	(647)	71,813	72,460	4,663	5,796	14.27

[a]Extender practice figures are for entire practice, rather than on a per-physician basis.
[b]Grant subsidy funds were excluded, but no attempt was made to remove the impact of the subsidies on cost.
[c]Includes outpatient hospital encounters.
[d]Not applicable.

$18,000 and $35,000. To gain some insight into some of the contributors to self-sufficiency, table 5-1 includes measures of office encounters per physician, total encounters per physician, average price per encounter, total costs per physician, and total revenues per physician for each practice.

Table 5-1 illustrates that net practice income per physician varies from a positive $60,000 to a loss of almost $65,000 per year. Thus, there is a variation of almost $125,000 in net practice income per physican per year among the eleven practices studied. Similarly, total revenue per practice physician varies from $39,800 to over $121,000, and total cost per physician varies from just over $40,000 to almost $122,000.[1] Primary-care encounters per physician (per year) range from 3,207 to 7,530, more than a factor-of-2 difference; total encounters range from 3,510 to 7,919; and average price per encounter varies from $10.90 to $18.55.

Clearly, even among only eleven practices, there is an extremely wide variation in self-sufficiency and in some of the factors that contribute to self-sufficiency. What are the key factors which determine the extent to which a practice can achieve self-sufficiency? We analyze the components of practice self-sufficiency. The revenues, costs, volume, prices, service mix, and collection rates of practices that are currently self-sufficient are compared with those that are not self-sufficient to analyze the relative importance of each of these elements.

Methodology

Extensive financial data were collected on eleven rural practices. Because of limitations in data collection and the difficulties inherent in assigning physician time to extender activities, both the sponsored and unsponsored extender practices were eliminated from this detailed analysis, leaving a total of nine practices for consideration.

The methodology was designed to standardize each practice in terms of a sole-proprietorship/partnership model, which enables comparisons of each practice relative to the income generated for the physician(s). This approach emphasizes the financial viability of each practice in terms of the amount of practice income available per physician, and it designates a practice as self-sufficient when the practice is able to generate a net income sufficient to maintain the physician(s) at the site. In this book, it was assumed that the practice net income in 1978 must be above $30,000 per physician for the physician to remain in practice in a rural area. The $30,000 figure was chosen to be the definer of self-sufficiency for a number of reasons. When questioned about the minimum acceptable income which would maintain them in rural areas, most physicians stated approximately $30,000. This was also observed by the research team; that is, viable practices tend to generate at least \$30,000 in net income per physician. Finally, this figure is approximately the opportunity cost of the physician's time, since she or he could elect to work for the NHSC or for another physician as a junior partner for about this salary level.

Three of the nine sites visited generated a net income (or service revenues in excess of costs) per physician of \$30,000 and are hereafter referred to as *currently self-sufficient*. One site yielded a \$20,000 net income to its physician; this practice is referred to in this discussion as "potentially self-sufficient."[2] Three other practices operated in a deficit position. These three, plus two others which generated a net income per physician of less than \$10,000, are termed in this discussion *non-self-sufficient*.

The following simple equations specify the relationships among the various factors which contribute to practice self-sufficiency:

$$\text{Net practice income} = \text{total revenues} - \text{total costs} \qquad (5.1)$$

where total costs do not include physician labor. Collections were used as the basis of revenue measurement for a variety of reasons discussed in chapter 4, under "Financial-Data Analysis."

Total collections equal the sum of the collections for each of the service centers of the practice, where the service centers in this analysis were ambulatory care, ancillary care, nursing-home care, and hospital care. For any of the service areas,

$$\text{Revenues} = \text{collections} = \text{price} \times \text{quantity} \times \text{collection rate} \qquad (5.2)$$

Furthermore, to analyze the profitability of a given service area, net contributions were calculated:

$$\text{Net contribution} = \text{collections} - \text{variable costs} \qquad (5.3)$$

The findings presented in the following sections should be interpreted as indicative of major trends and highlights relative to rural-practice self-sufficiency, and not as definitive statements about all rural practices under all conditions. The sample size used in this book is very small and was chosen, as discussed in chapter 4, by a process of nomination and selection, rather than randomly. Only as far as these sampled practices reflect rural practices as a whole can the findings presented here be generalized to all rural practices. Although one should be cautious in interpreting the important patterns found among the currently self-sufficient, potentially self-sufficient, and non-self-sufficient practices, they do appear to be consistent with the findings of other researchers. We believe that the major findings are likely to be substantiated in future, more extensive research efforts.

General Findings Related to Degrees of Self-Sufficiency

Table 5-2 separates the practices according to the self-sufficiency status. Revenues, costs, and income per physician and per encounter for the practices are presented. We refer to the averages for the group, but discuss the specific practice data when there is wide variation within a group.

As a group, self-sufficient practices generated a total revenue per physician nearly twice (180 percent) that of the non-self-sufficient practices, a difference of $43,764. On the other hand, average total cost per physician of the self-sufficient practices is about $24,000 lower, a reduction of about 30 percent. Although total costs are substantially lower in self-sufficient practices, the effect of additional revenues is even stronger; and the result is that total revenues are more important than total costs in determining net income per physician. As can be seen from the individual practice data, none of the non-self-sufficient practices (E through I) had revenues exceeding $58,000. Thus, their revenues were at least $20,000 less than the lowest revenue per physician ($76,960) of the self-sufficient practices.

On a per-encounter basis, revenues on average are roughly equivalent in self-sufficient and non-self-sufficient practices ($13.08 versus $11.80), while the average cost of the non-self-sufficient practice ($16.02) is over twice that of the self-sufficient ($7.32). What causes this reversal in the relationship between revenues and costs as we move from total to per-unit measure? In going from total costs to average costs, the effect of volume has been incorporated. Therefore, the lower volume of the non-self-sufficient practice results in their having lower total revenues and higher average costs per encounter.

Findings Related to Revenues

In determining the difference in revenues between self-sufficient and non-self-sufficient practices, total encounters appear to be a much more important factor than average price per encounter or the collection rate. But among those with incomes in excess of $30,000 per physician, higher prices per encounter account for much of the variation in income. The practice with the highest net income has an average price $2.50 to $4.50 higher than the other two self-sufficient practices. The price effect is discussed in more detail later. Also, among the non-self-sufficient practices, those with very high cost had the greatest deficits.

Table 5-3 presents encounters per physician, average price per encounter, and collection rate for practices at different levels of self-sufficiency. The differences between self-sufficient and non-self-sufficient practices on the dimensions of average price per encounter ($15.40 versus $14.20) and collection rate (85.6 versus 82.4 percent) are not great. There is

Table 5-2
Revenues, Costs, and Income per Physician and per Encounter for Practices with Varying Degrees of Self-Sufficiency
(dollars)

Degree of Self-Sufficiency	Total Revenue per Physician	Average Revenue per Encounter	Total Cost per Physician	Average Cost per Encounter	Net Gain/(Loss) per Encounter	Average Net Income per Physician
Currently self-sufficient (*n* = 3)	98,642	13.08	55,173	7.32	5.76	43,468
Practice A (Unsponsored solo physician, hospital in town)	97,607	12.88	64,077	8.45	4.43	33,530
Practice B (Unsponsored group practice, hospital in town)	121,358	15.32	61,095	7.71	7.61	60,263
Practice C (Unsponsored group practice, 10 miles from hospital)	76,960	11.04	40,347	5.79	5.25	36,612
Potentially self-sufficient (*n* = 1)						
Practice D (Sponsored solo physician, 20 + miles from hospital)	93,319	12.25	72,904	9.57	2.68	20,415
Not self-sufficient (*n* = 5)	54,878	11.80	79,165	16.02	(4.22)	(24,287)
Practice E (Sponsored group practice, hospital in town)	50,707	11.98	40,778	9.64	2.34	9,929
Practice F (Sponsored group practice with two satellite clinics)	54,811	10.98	92,956	18.63	(7.65)	(38,145)

Practice G (Unsponsored solo physician, 20+ miles from hospital)	57,942	15.19	51,227	13.43	1.76	6,715
Practice H (Sponsored solo physician, hospital in town)	57,520	8.04	121,966	17.04	(9.00)	(64,446)
Practice I (Sponsored group practice, 10 miles from hospital)	53,408	12.83	88,898	21.36	(8.53)	(35,490)

Table 5-3
Total Encounters per Physician, Average Price per Encounter, and Collection Rate for Practices with Varying Degrees of Self-Sufficiency

Degree of Self-Sufficiency	Total Encounters per Physician	Average Price per Encounter ($)	Collection Rate (%)
Currently self-sufficient (n = 3)	7,491	15.40	85.6
Practice A (Unsponsored solo physician, hospital in town)	7,581	15.66	82.1
Practice B (Unsponsored group practice, hospital in town)	7,919	18.55	82.5
Practice C (Unsponsored group practice, 10 miles from hospital)	6,971	11.98	92.1
Potentially self-sufficient (n = 1)			
Practice D (Sponsored solo physician, 20+ miles from hospital)	7,620	13.44	91.0
Not self-sufficient (n = 5)	4,871	14.20	82.4
Practice E (Sponsored group practice, hospital in town)	4,231	14.10	85.0
Practice F (Sponsored group practice with two satellite clinics)	4,990	14.76	74.4
Practice G (Unsponsored solo physician, 20+ miles from hospital)	3,814	16.19	93.8
Practice H (Sponsored solo physician, hospital in town)	7,158	10.90	73.7
Practice I (Sponsored group practice, 10 miles from hospital)	4,162	15.05	85.2

a major difference, however, in the encounter rate per physician (7,491 versus 4,871): Practices that are self-sufficient provide 54 percent more patient encounters per physician. Even if the collection rate and average price per encounter were equalized for both types of practices, the non-self-sufficient practices would increase their total revenues per physician only from 56 to 63 percent of the revenues generated by the self-sufficient practices.

Practice H, the sponsored solo practice, is the one exception. If its collection rate rose to that of the practice with which it was matched, its income would have increased by 11 percent, to $64,000. The lower prices of the non-self-sufficient practice mostly reflect the sliding-fee schedule of the practices and their greater ambulatory-care orientation, both of which are related to their being sponsored practices.

Importance of Encounters

If encounters per physician were equalized between the self-sufficient and non-self-sufficient practices, the difference in total revenues per physician would be *only about 11 percent*. Of this 11 percent, the average price per encounter accounts for about 7 percent, and the collection rate accounts for about 4 percent.

Further insights on the nature of the encounters are gained when encounters are distributed across the four major service centers of primary-care practices. Table 5-4 lists ambulatory, ancillary, nursing-home, and hospital encounters per physician for the practices according to level of self-sufficiency.

The most striking difference in encounters between self-sufficient and non-self-sufficient practices occurs in hospital care (2,257 versus 771 encounters per physician). Hospital encounters account for 30 percent of all encounters for the self-sufficient practices and only 16 percent in the non-self-sufficient practices. While self-sufficient practices provide 25 percent more office encounters, they conduct 193 percent more hospital encounters. Nursing-home encounters are not significant for either group.

Practice H appears to be an exception, once again. The hospital encounters of this practice (1,689) are much higher than the other, non-self-sufficient practices. This number, which had to be estimated from patient files, may be on the high side. (There was a hospital in the town which the physician used regularly. Nevertheless, the hospital administrator did not believe the physician admitted patients as often as the other physicians who practiced in town. Revenue-collection data could not be used since the practice did not always bill for hospital care.)

A practice that offers more services can generate more revenue from patients. A wide scope of services also is considered to be an important ele-

Table 5-4
Ambulatory, Ancillary, Nursing-Home, and Hospital Encounters per Physician for Practices of Varying Degrees of Self-Sufficiency

Degree of Self-Sufficiency	Service Center			
	Ambulatory Office Encounters per Physician	Ancillary In-House Procedures per Physician	Nursing Home Nursing-Home Encounters per Physician	Hospital Hospital Encounters Per Physician
Currently self-sufficient (n = 3)	5,084	1,578	149	2,257
Practice A (Unsponsored solo physician, hospital in town)	5,193	1,584	0	2,388
Practice B (Unsponsored group practice, hospital in town)	4,901	1,534	81	2,937
Practice C (Unsponsored group practice, 10 miles from hospital)	5,158	1,617	367	1,447
Potentially self-sufficient (n = 1)				
Practice D (Sponsored solo physician, 20+ miles from hospital)	7,530	2,629	90	0[a]
Not self-sufficient (n = 5)	4,069	972	31	771
Practice E (Sponsored group practice, hospital in town)	3,454	0	100	678
Practice F (Sponsored group practice with two satellite clinics)	4,248	1,164	0	742

Practice G (Unsponsored solo physician, 20+ miles from hospital)	3,207	610	55	552
Practice H (Sponsored solo physician, hospital in town)	5,469	1,730	0	1,689[b]
Practice I (Sponsored group practice, 10 miles from hospital)	3,966	1,357	0	196

[a]The potentially self-sufficient practice is a sponsored, solo-physician practice, located over 20 miles from the nearest hospital, which does not offer any hospital-based services.

[b]Estimated.

ment in practice building. Patients expect their family physicians to treat them for a wide variety of conditions, and the capacity to provide a wide range of services helps establish patient loyalty. For example, ancillary procedures allow a physician to give more sophisticated care and at the same time generate additional income. (The issue of overuse of technology in terms of medical necessity was not analyzed. The positive findings about the value of technology are in terms of financial viability only.)

The encounter data are translated into revenues for the same services in table 5-5. The group averages illustrate that while self-sufficient practices generate higher revenues in each service center, the difference in hospital-care revenues ($28,028) is greater than the difference of all the other service centers combined. Further, self-sufficient rural practices derive a much higher proportion of their total revenue from hospitalization (38 versus 18 percent). As can be seen from the averages as well as the individual practices, the difference in revenue from ambulatory care is quite small. Three of the non-self-sufficient practices have incomes that exceed $40,000 and are just a few thousand less than those of the self-sufficient practice. For each of the service centers, a few additional comments are warranted.

Hospital Care. The value of hospital services to rural-practice viability is underscored by additional evidence gained through interviews with physicians. The availability of hospital services is important in the rural physician's decision of where to practice, in providing comprehensive care that helps establish patient loyalty, and in contributing to practice income. The physicians perceived the following considerations to be important regarding the availability of hospital services:

1. Hospital privileges were essential to their practices because they improve diagnostic capability and continuity of care, as well as favorably contribute to the physician's own sense of happiness and interest in practicing medicine.
2. The availability of hospital services was important from the patient's perspective. It was noted that patients do not like to be referred to another physician for hospital care, that such a referral reduces patient confidence, worsens continuity of care, and in the end loses patients for the practice.
3. The one physician without a hospital practice (located 23 miles from a hospital) had learned to refer patients needing hospitalization only to specialists who would send them back to him for primary care. In addition, at the time of the research, this physician was preparing to go into partnership with a surgeon in order to be able to establish a hospital component of sufficient size to be economically feasible for the practice.[3]

Table 5-5
Revenues per Physician and Percentage of Total Revenues by Service Center for Practices of Varying Degrees of Self-Sufficiency

Degree of Self-Sufficiency	Ambulatory Care	Ancillary Care	Nursing-Home Care	Hospital Care	Total Revenues
	Revenues per Physician (Percentage of Total Revenues) for:				
Currently self-sufficient (n = 3)	$46,488 (47.1%)	$12,798 (13.0%)	$1,550 (1.6%)	$37,805 (38.3%)	$98,641 (100%)
Practice A (Unsponsored solo physician, hospital in town)	48,089 (49%)	12,183 (12%)	0 (—)	37,335 (38%)	97,607 (100%)
Practice B (Unsponsored group practice, hospital in town)	47,790 (39%)	16,056 (13%)	752 (1%)	56,761 (47%)	121,359 (100%)
Practice C (Unsponsored group practice, 10 miles from hospital)	43,584 (57%)	10,157 (13%)	3,901 (5%)	19,318 (25%)	76,960 (100%)
Potentially self-sufficient (n = 1)					
Practice D (Sponsored solo physician, 20+ miles from hospital)	70,524 (75.6%)	21,536 (23.1%)	1,259 (1.3%)	0 (0%)	93,319 (100%)
Not self-sufficient (n = 5)	37,841 (68.9%)	6,873 (12.5%)	387 (0.7%)	9,777 (17.8%)	54,878 (100%)
Practice E (Sponsored group practice, hospital in town)	42,450 (84%)	0 (—)	1,060 (2%)	7,198 (14%)	50,708 (100%)
Practice F (Sponsored group practice with two satellite clinics)	40,971 (75%)	7,113 (13%)	0 (—)	6,720 (12%)	54,804 (100%)

Table 5-5 *(continued)*

Degree of Self-Sufficiency	Revenues per Physician (Percentage of Total Revenues) for:				
	Ambulatory Care	Ancillary Care	Nursing-Home Care	Hospital Care	Total Revenues
Practice G (Unsponsored solo physician, 20+ miles from hospital)	$41,110 (71%)	$6,522 (11%)	$866 (1%)	$9,444 (16%)	$57,942 (100%)
Practice H (Sponsored solo physician, hospital in town)	29,127 (51%)	5,766 (10%)	0 —	22,627	57,520
Practice I (Sponsored group practice, 10 miles from hospital)	35,545 (67%)	14,966 (28%)	0 —	2,897 (5%)	53,408 (100%)

4. Emergency-room contact with patients is an important source of new clientele for the practice.

In summary, the availability of hospital services is important to a rural practice because it allows a physician to provide a more comprehensive scope of services and because of its income potential. With respect to net practice income, the hospital portion of a practice turns out to be very significant since the associated costs are so small. Overall, the contribution of hospital services to the profitability of the practice depends on sufficient volume to justify the opportunity costs of the physician's time. The solo practitioner who had a potentially self-sufficient practice argued that since he was over 20 miles from the hospital, it was uneconomical for him to see his patients in the hospital since it would take so much time away from a busy office practice.

The practice with the highest net income per physician, which was the only practice with per-physician net income above $40,000, had the highest ratio of hospital to total encounters and conducted the most surgical procedures. The high income of this practice, which had a hospital nearby, can be traced to its hospital practice. Whether the greater use of the hospital resulted in a higher or lower quality of health care for their patients was not considered in this research on financial viability.

Ambulatory Care. Office visits, especially for primary-care-oriented physicians, represent the majority of the provider's direct contact with patients. Table 5-4 illustrates that both currently self-sufficient and non-self-sufficient practices provide more than 4,200 office encounters per physician per year. (The encounters per physician encompass all those done at the practice. Therefore, if a nurse or physician extender conducted visits, the number of encounters per physician shown in this table would be higher than those done by the physician alone.) In terms of revenue per physician, self-sufficient practices generate about $10,000 more from ambulatory care.

It appears that a better predictor of rural-practice self-sufficiency may be total encounters per physician. Table 5-3 indicates that self-sufficient practices provide 7,491 total encounters per physician while non-self-sufficient practices provide only 4,871. The minimum level of encounters necessary for self-sufficiency, however, will depend also on the practice's service-delivery mix. Since hospital and nursing-home encounters tend to yield higher incomes to the practice because of higher prices and lower variable costs, practices with vigorous hospital and nursing-home components will require lower total encounters per physician to achieve financial viability. The potentially self-sufficient practice had over 7,500 office encounters. Practices with a smaller level of encounters were more profitable largely because they provided hospital care.

Ancillary Care. Table 5-6 presents four measures of ancillary activities. It is apparent from this table that self-sufficient practices conduct more laboratory tests and x-rays per physician than non-self-sufficient practices. However, when they are standardized for the number of office encounters, it can be seen that in both cases approximately 25 percent of the patients received laboratory tests. In none of the practices were laboratory tests given to more than 35 percent of those who came to the office. The higher patient volume of the self-sufficient practices allows them to distribute the fixed cost over a larger number of tests. Nevertheless, laboratory tests were not found profitable even for self-sufficient rural practices because of the associated high variable costs. Table 5-7 lists the average profit or loss from internal laboratories, external laboratories, and x-rays for four practices where these factors could be isolated. Only x-rays are profitable for self-sufficient practices; laboratory procedures tend to lose money for all types of practices. For all three categories combined, the two self-sufficient practices show a profit of about $500, and the two non-self-sufficient show a loss of about $8,000.

This finding is contrary to the conventional wisdom in the field, which assumes that ancillary procedures are profitable for most practices. A reason may be that administrative costs usually are not allocated to this category of services. This is done because it is argued that administrative costs are fixed. If administrative costs are excluded entirely, a different picture does emerge. As shown in table 5-7, a profit of about $5,700 would result for the two self-sufficient practices, and the loss for the two non-self-sufficient practices would drop to around $700. Since administrative costs are raised by the amount of laboratory volume, the latter figures exceed any reasonable estimation of the profitability of ancillary activities.

In discussions with the administrators and physicians at the rural practices, with the exception of those associated with the physician-extender practices, it was found that ancillary services were not designed to be a source of profits, but rather were priced to cover costs.

Nursing-Home Care. Tables 5-4 and 5-5 illustrate that nursing-home care is not important to the rural practices studied, in terms of either encounters or revenue generated. This is a somewhat surprising result. It may be that the practices were still too young to have a significant patient load in nursing homes. Nevertheless, the physicians did not view the nursing home as an important profit center.

Findings Related to Collection Rate

Table 5-3 demonstrates that the collection rate for self-sufficient practices averages 85.6 percent, while the non-self-sufficient practices average 82.4

Table 5-6
Measures of Ancillary Activity in 1978 for Practices of Varying Degrees of Self-Sufficiency

Degree of Self-Sufficiency	Laboratory Visits per Physician	Laboratory Visits as a Percentage of Office Visits	In-House X-ray Visits per Physician	Laboratory Procedures per Patient Receiving Laboratory Services
Currently self-sufficient (n = 3)	1,359	26.7	219	1.12
Practice A (Unsponsored solo physician, hospital in town)	1,227	23.6	357	
Practice B (Unsponsored group practice, hospital in town)	1,233	25.2	301	
Practice C (Unsponsored group practice, 10 miles from hospital)	1,617	31.3	0	
Potentially self-sufficient (n = 1)				
Practice D (Sponsored solo physician, 20 + miles from hospital)	2,221	29.5	408	1.52
Not self-sufficient (n = 5)	931	22.7	41	1.67
Practice E (Sponsored group practice, hospital in town)	0[a]	0[a]	0	
Practice F (Sponsored group practice with two satellite clinics)	1,086	25.6	78	

Table 5-6 *(continued)*

Degree of Self-Sufficiency	Laboratory Visits per Physician	Laboratory Visits as a Percentage of Office Visits	In-House X-ray Visits per Physician	Laboratory Procedures per Patient Receiving Laboratory Services
Practice G (Unsponsored solo physician, 20+ miles from hospital)	519	16.2	91	
Practice H (Sponsored solo physician, hospital in town)	1,694	31.0	36	
Practice I (Sponsored group practice, 10 miles from hospital)	1,357	34.2	0	

[a]All tests were done in the adjacent hospital.

Table 5-7
Average Profit/(Loss) due to Ancillary Activities for Practices of Varying Degrees of Self-Sufficiency
(dollars)

Degree of Self-Sufficiency	Internal Laboratory (1)	External Laboratory (2)	X-ray (3)	Total of (1), (2), and (3) with Administration Costs	Total of (1), (2), and (3) without Administration Costs
Self-sufficient[a] (n = 2)	(231)	(2,151)	2,892	510	5,665
Not self-sufficient (n = 2)	(3,075)	(3,502)	(1,470)	(8,047)	731

[a]Includes potentially self-sufficient.

percent, a difference of only about 3 percent and too small an average to significantly affect self-sufficiency. Two of the non-self-sufficient practices, both sponsored, did have a much lower collection rate (74 percent). In one of these sites, the physician decided how aggressively to seek collection on an ad hoc basis, while at the other there was a written policy with a sequential follow-up procedure. At both practices, the notion of treating the poor was felt deeply and could explain the lower collection rate. Raising their collection rates by 10 percentage points would reduce the deficits of this practice by less than $10,000, still leaving them with substantial shortfalls.

Findings Related to Price

Three major factors influence the average price per encounter realized by a rural practice: service mix, or the relative amounts of services offered (for example, hospital and office visits); the intensity and complexity of the office or hospital encounter; and the prevailing charge structure. The difference in the average price per encounter between the self-sufficient and non-self-sufficient practices on average is less than 8 percent ($15.40 versus $14.20); however, this small difference in averages masks the variation which exists. For the self-sufficient practices, the variation in average price is about 55 percent, from $11.98 to $18.55, and for the non-self-sufficient a somewhat lower variation existed, from $10.90 to $16.19. The following sections explore the reasons for differences in the average price among the self-sufficient practices.

Relationship between Average Price per Encounter and Services Mix. In an earlier discussion relating to scope of services, it was shown that self-sufficient practices derive substantially higher revenues from hospital visits. Since the average price for a hospital visit usually exceeds that of an office visit, it follows that a higher average price per encounter exists in practices that hospitalize more. On average, the self-sufficient practices also charged more for hospital visits, suggesting that they do more complex procedures, for example, surgery. Table 5-8 presents data which break down the difference in average price per encounter among the three self-sufficient practices and the group average for the non-self-sufficient practices per encounter according to the volume and price for hospital care, amount of ancillary procedures, and prevailing charge structure.

The volume of hospital encounters explains the difference in average price per encounter between the two groups of practices and the much higher average price ($18.55) of practice B. The ancillary effect, or the intensity of an office visit, is not a major factor in accounting for differences in average price per encounter. The figures in the final column suggest that

Table 5-8
Hospital and Ancillary Effect on Average Price per Encounter
(dollars)

| | Average Price per Encounter | | | Difference Caused by: | | | | |
| | Self-Sufficient Practices | Non-self-Sufficient Practices, Weighted Average | Difference | Hospital Effect | | Ancillary Effect | | |
				Volume	Pricing	Volume	Pricing	Other
Practice A	15.66	14.36	1.30	3.27	0.09	(0.21)	0	(1.85)
Practice B	18.55	14.36	4.19	5.46	0.70	(0.40)	0.74	(2.31)
Practice C	11.98	14.36	(2.38)	0.97	(0.55)	0.02	(0.58)	(2.24)

self-sufficient practices charged less for a basic office visit and conducted proportionately fewer of these visits.

The self-sufficient practices appear able to charge these lower office rates because of the strong positive contribution of hospital volume toward average price per encounter. One might infer from these data that the self-sufficient practices are able to use hospital revenues to cross-subsidize ambulatory care. In terms of practice utilization and income, such cross-subsidization makes good business sense. Since patients often have to pay out of their own pockets for office visits while hospitalizations are insured, this cross-subsidization in prices should work to increase the total demand for care by the patients of the practice.

Importance of Urban and Rural Reimbursement-Rate Differentials. In three of the six states visited, an urban-rural Medicare reimbursement-rate differential existed, with rural rates always lower than urban rates. Table 5-9 summarizes the prevailing charges for Medicare in the six states visited.

In the most extreme, but not unrepresentative, case (South), the total billings of the sponsored practice would have been 20 percent higher, or $15,000, if rural reimbursement rates had been raised to urban levels (and if the entire practice's charge structure followed the Medicare pattern). For the Midwest sponsored practice, the annual revenues would be increased by $5,500 if the urban rates had been applied. Change in total revenue of these magnitudes may not raise a non-self-sufficient practice to a self-sufficient level, but they would constitute a significant increase in practice net income since no additional costs would ensue.

This effect is further scrutinized in the Appendix where a linear-programming model is used to simulate a rural medical practice 30 miles from a hospital. The model illustrates that substituting urban for rural reimbursement rates increases the annual net income by 25 percent, but does not change the optimal mix of services the practice should provide to maximize income. As hospitalization rates of the practice are increased in the simulation, the impact of urban rates on net income becomes more pronounced. This is because the differentials for hospital services are the largest. (See the Appendix for a more complete discussion of the implications of substituting urban for rural reimbursement rates.)

Findings Related to Cost

The wide variation in the cost structures of the rural practices studied was partially illustrated in table 5-1, which presented total costs per physician.

Table 5-10 divides the costs into nonphysician medical labor, ad-

Table 5-9
Urban-Rural Reimbursement-Rate Comparisons for the Six States Visited

Procedure	South		Mid-Atlantic		Midwest[a]			West Statewide Rate	Southwest Statewide Rate	Northwest Statewide Rate
	Rural Rate	Urban Rate	Rural Rate	Urban Rate	Rural Rate 1	Rural Rate 2	Urban Rate			
Average for office visits	10.05	12.25	16.43	18.80	14.56	15.75	15.64	16.72	17.30	12.25
Average for hospital visits	13.15	16.55	25.10	35.10	17.60	18.30	19.75	25.10	27.50	19.50
Average x-ray	27.14	28.14	30.20	30.40	23.20	25.20	24.00	34.24	30.40	14.90
Average laboratory	5.86	6.41	5.68	5.94	6.00	6.27	6.05	6.61	5.04	5.47

[a]In this state the rates paid varied by county. The rates shown are for the rural counties in which the two practices operated.

Table 5-10
Nonphysician Medical Labor, Administrative Costs, Plant Costs, and Total Costs per Physician and per Encounter for Practices of Varying Degrees of Self-Sufficiency
(dollars)

Degree of Self-Sufficiency	Nonphysician Medical Labor		Administrative Costs		Plant Costs		Total Costs	
	Per Physician	*Per Total Encounter*	*Per Physician*	*Per Total Encounter*	*Per Physician*	*Per Total Encounter*	*Per Physician*	*Per Total Encounter*
Currently self-sufficient (*n* = 3)	12,362	1.65	16,290	2.17	18,590	2.47	55,173	7.32
Practice A (Unsponsored solo physician, hospital in town)	11,150	1.47	16,545	2.18	29,203	3.86	64,077	8.45
Practice B (Unsponsored group practice, hospital in town)	10,266	1.30	25,126	3.17	15,214	1.92	61,095	7.71
Practice C (Unsponsored group practice, 10 miles from hospital)	15,671	2.24	7,200	1.03	11,352	1.62	40,347	5.79
Potentially self-sufficient (*n* = 1)								
Practice D (Sponsored solo physician, 20+ miles from hospital)	8,075	1.06	23,954	3.15	17,941	2.35	72,904	9.56
Not self-sufficient (*n* = 5)	17,126	2.29	26,554	3.54	19,460	2.60	79,165	16.25
Practice E (Sponsored group practice, hospital in town)	4,576	1.08	15,736	3.71	14,877	3.52	40,778	9.64
Practice F (Sponsored group practice with two satellite clinics)	24,026	4.81	37,909	7.59	19,125	3.84	92,956	18.63

Practice G (Unsponsored solo physician, 20+ miles from hospital)	11,426	3.00	17,911	4.69	14,843	3.89	51,227	13.43
Practice H (Sponsored solo physician, hospital in town)	24,647	3.44	31,589	4.41	25,174	3.51	121,966	17.04
Practice I (Sponsored group practice, 10 miles from hospital)	20,953	5.03	29,627	7.12	23,283	5.60	88,898	21.36

ministrative costs, and plant costs on a per-physician and per-encounter basis for practices of varying degrees of self-sufficiency.

Whereas the average charge for the self-sufficient practices exceeded that of the non-self-sufficient practices by $1.20, the average cost per encounter was $8.70 less than, or 55 percent of, the average cost for the non-self-sufficient counterparts.

Some of the higher costs shown in table 5-1 are associated with outreach and other nonmedical services. These are not included in the three cost categories of table 5-10. When these are deleted, the dollar difference in cost narrows to about $6.70. For all the three cost categories presented in table 5-10—nonphysician labor, administrative, and plant costs—the average for non-self-sufficient practices exceeds that for the self-sufficient practices. The greatest difference is administrative costs, and for these costs all the self-sufficient practices have lower costs than any in the non-self-sufficient category.

If we turn to the other cost categories, in two instances the individual practice costs overlap. First, the nonphysician labor cost of practice E was the least for any practice, self-sufficient or not. Second, the plant cost for practice A exceeded those of two of the non-self-sufficient practices. There are reasons for these discrepancies. In practice E, the physicians were located at the hospital and had a very low patient volume. These factors minimized the need for a nurse. The high plant costs of practice A resulted from his moving into a newly built and large facility that had been left behind by a physician who moved out of the area. His payments for equipment were particularly out of line. The other reason for the higher cost was that he was a solo physician, and therefore he suffered from diseconomies of scale. Obviously, the sample is too small to make any precise judgments about the impact of scale, but it does appear that diseconomies are more important in terms of capital than labor inputs and costs. The solo physician had a reception area, laboratory space, and often an x-ray room similar to the two- and three-person practice. Also, the number of examining rooms per physicians seems to fall as the number of physicians in the group increases. One reason for this observation is that it is unlikely that peak examining-room needs of all physicians will occur simultaneously. Therefore, the optimum number of examining rooms is less than the multiple of the number of physicians. These costs are discussed in chapter 6.

While the scale factor is important, the critical reason for the difference in total cost per encounter is volume. The non-self-sufficient practices are operating with underutilized medical and administrative personnel as well as physical space.

Net Contribution of Various Service Centers

A major effort of this book is to identify the services which produce the net income of rural medical practices. To do this, the non-physician medical personnel and administrative costs associated with three service centers of medical practices—office, nursing home, and hospital care—were identified and compared to revenues. The differences are calculated as practice net contributions and are presented in table 5-11.

Table 5-11, which is the most revealing of the data sets included, shows that the ambulatory-care revenues generated by the non-self-sufficient practices were not even meeting their medical and administrative costs, as reflected in their negative contributions for the office portion of their practice. This indicates the pattern of overstaffing of both medical and administrative personnel just discussed. For the self-sufficient practices, the office yields about $27,500 in net contributions. The difference in the net contributions from office contributions for self-sufficient and non-self-sufficient practices ($37,686) is primarily a function of differences in costs rather than in volume. As was shown earlier, the difference in office encounters (5,084 versus 4,069) results in a difference of only about $13,000 in office revenues. Therefore, costs account for two-thirds of the difference in the net contributions of the office.

Nursing-home income is insignificant for both the self-sufficient and non-self-sufficient practices. And it has been shown in table 5-7 that laboratory tests are not a profit center for the practices for which financial data were available. This is due to the high variable costs associated with providing these services.

Table 5-11
Net Contributions by Service Center for Practices of Varying Degrees of Self-Sufficiency
(dollars)

Degree of Self-Sufficiency	Service Center Net Contribution per Physician		
	Office	*Nursing Home*	*Hospital*
Currently self-sufficient (n = 3)	27,407	1,371	33,280
Practice A	29,731	0	33,002
Practice B	26,163	533	48,783
Practice C	26,328	3,581	18,056
Potentially self-sufficient (n = 1)			
Practice D	37,308	1,048	0
Not self-sufficient (n = 5)	10,279	265	5,184
Practice E	19,442	688	4,677
Practice F	(20,691)	0	1,651
Practice G	13,568	634	7,356
Practice H	(49,890)	0	10,618
Practice I	(13,826)	0	1,620

Note: See table 5-10 for practice descriptions.

There is a large difference in the hospital contributions realized, but this is attributable primarily to volume (2,257 versus 771 hospital encounters per physician) rather than to differences in costs. For self-sufficient practices, the hospital is a very profitable service center, since contributions are 90 percent of revenues (while office contributions are only 47 percent of revenues). This is because little in the way of additional costs, other than those associated with the physician's time, occur when a hospital encounter takes place. Total revenues from hospitalization for this group were $37,805 (table 5-5). Thus, only $4,600 is lost because of associated costs. For the office portion of their practices, the comparable figures are $46,488 and $27,407, or a drop of about $19,000 because of associated costs. The importance of hospitalization to net practice income is further inhibited by the variation in net contribution among self-sufficient practices. While their contributions from the office are virtually identical, it is the hospital which allows practices to earn substantially in excess of the self-sufficiency level of $30,000. Also, in analyzing the individual data for non-self-sufficient practices, it is evident that if Practices E and G had had hospital revenues comparable to the self-sufficient practices, then they would have earned sufficient net incomes.

Summary Comments on Practice Self-Sufficiency

On average, the revenues generated by the non-self-sufficient practices from their offices were not even meeting their medical and administrative costs. On the other hand, self-sufficient practices realized close to $30,000 in net contributions from their office practices alone. Since the plant and other fixed costs per physician for these practices are, on average, about $18,500, it seems reasonable to argue that a typical rural practice providing about 4,000 to 5,000 office visits and no hospitalization would generate approximately $10,000 to $15,000 in net income. The break-even point (excluding physician income) appears to be between 3,000 and 3,500 visits depending on fixed costs. Above this level, physician net income becomes positive and rises with encounters. This observation is supported by the potentially self-sufficient practice site that shows a net income of little over $20,000 from over 7,500 office encounters. The high costs of this solo practice made the break-even output level somewhat higher.

These net-income findings have considerable importance for the NHSC program. If NHSC physicians providing 4,200 office visits (which is the target for the program) generate only $10,000 to $15,000 for physician income, then becoming a private physician in the community will have little appeal. The findings indicate that a hospital practice is a necessity if rural physicians are to earn net income in the vicinity of $30,000 with 4,000 to

5,000 office visits.[4] Five thousand office visits will generate a net income of only about $15,000. If the physician had 1,000 hospital visits, the practice would be able to earn another $15,000. The higher profitability from the hospital visits reflects the higher fees paid for hospital visits and the insignificant practice costs attached to hospital visits. Physicians' net incomes will be even higher if they perform surgical procedures at the hospital. Of all the practices visited, only one had physician incomes in excess of $37,000. This practice had 490 hospital admissions per physician, or about one for every ten clinic encounters per physician. Of these, 25 percent were surgical cases, and they generated about 55 percent of the practice's hospital revenue. An understanding of the importance of surgery by the practices themselves is evidenced by the recent actions taken in two practices. In one of the non-self-sufficient practices, a new administrator who was an employee of a private management-consulting firm, stated that once he recruited a general surgeon to the practice, it would become self-sufficient. Another private, self-sufficient practice had sought an orthopedic surgeon as its third member.

These findings provide clues as to how a rural physician must provide care under today's fee-for-service system in order to earn an income sufficient to keep the provider in a rural area.

First, the physician must have a sufficient office-practice volume—hypothetically 100 patients per week. Of the 100 visits, five or ten will have to be admitted to the hospital. If 5 percent, or 250 per year, were hospitalized and the physician provided eight visits per patient, or 2,000 visits per year, the physician would earn close to $40,000. Incomes in excess of that require a higher hospitalization or visit per admission rate. Given the time constraints on the practitioners and the existing reimbursement rates, the easiest way to improve average income per hospital encounter is to perform surgery.

High hospitalization rates and the performance of surgical procedures will be financially beneficial to the practice. Whether this will be beneficial to the patients of the practice depends in part on whether a larger proportion of their medical expenditures are being secured by this practice or whether they will be expending more on medical care in toto. Even if we assume the best, which is that their expenditures are shifted to the rural practice, the net effect on the total system is likely to be an increase in costs and subsequently higher health-care expenditures. This is because more self-contained medical practices will mean increased total capacity. The question surrounding quality remains: Are the rural providers equally competent to provide the care? And, if they are not, are the convenience benefits to the patient more than offset by the poorer quality of care? These important issues lie beyond this book, but not beyond the concerns of policymakers.

Notes

1. The costs that ensue from grant programs are included in these numbers, even when the purpose is not to provide medical care. In the detailed analyses on costs, those not related to the provision of medical care were included.

2. This physician was preparing to convert to a private practice, and he was using his available income to purchase supplies and equipment. For this physician, if the prices charged were increased slightly or if he had charged for hospital visits he was making, the practice would have had a net income of over $30,000.

3. This practice is analyzed in depth in the Appendix, where a linear mathematical model of the practice is developed to gauge the effect of altering certain key factors. This model shows that if the practice has a moderate hospitalization component (three hospital encounters per day, five days per week), its net income will fall because of the practice's distance from the hospital.

4. A similar economic profile of a rural physician from North Carolina appeared in the January 27, 1979, issue of *Medical Economics*. This physician's net income from his medical practice was $24,050. The physician did not provide hospital care, but did operate his own pharmacy.

Performance of Sponsored and Unsponsored Rural Medical Practices

In the last chapter, the contributors to financial self-sufficiency of a practice are identified. This chapter examines and describes the dominant financial and operating characteristics associated with sponsorship.

Matched pairs of sponsored and unsponsored rural medical practices were selected in order to distinguish the particular effects of outside sponsorship on the manner in which the practice develops and is managed and the way in which care is delivered. Over time, it was realized that sponsorship must be separated from self-sufficiency in order to identify how sponsorship contributes to or hinders self-sufficiency.

The distinction between current and past sources of support is important here, for all eleven of the practice studies were recipients of outside support at some point.[1] For those practices categorized as private or unsponsored in this study, earlier support took the form of donated land and buildings; low-interest or noncollateral bank loans for office facilities, equipment, homes, and practice vehicles; and initial NHSC site sponsorship. The fact that today's private practices were yesterday's sponsored sites may be one indication of the intense financial challenges faced by rural practitioners who seek to establish a new practice. What are the critical differences between those practices which grow out of sponsorship to become viable and self-sufficient and those which remain dependent on external support over time? Although this is not a longitudinal analysis, comparison of five matched sets of sponsored and unsponsored practices allows for the identification of patterns of behavior which differentiate the practices.

Effects of Sponsorship

The dynamics of practice development and achievement of self-sufficiency can be influenced in three major ways by an outside sponsor. First, outside funding to a community for the establishment or continuing support of a medical practice could represent a solution to any of several nonmedical problems. Social, political, and economic concerns may govern such decisions. For example, a religious order may seek to expand its membership to meet a perceived need for health service in a specific community. County officials may foresee political gains from establishing a medical practice in a given geographic area. Local business leaders could view the establishment of a medical practice as an economic venture—a way to bring into a community other related firms, for example, a drug store, dentist, nursing home.

The financial implications for the medical practice which is established for such nonmedical motives usually are not fully considered. The practice may not have the necessary incentives to build the patient volume adequate to achieve self-sufficiency. Moreover, the location of the practice may be a poor one. For instance, if it is not placed within a "medical trade center," if it is too small to provide a comprehensive range of services, or if it is located too close to other established medical practices, a practice may not become financially viable.

Second, if the funding objectives of the grantor extend beyond the simple provision of medical care to local residents, then the practice may be structured to accommodate these broader objectives. On the cost side, sponsors may mandate certain modes of production or administrative procedures, for example, with the imposition of staffing ratios, staffing patterns, or the requirement that the practice install a full-time administrator. Moreover, an outside sponsor may also demand the provision of certain (uninsured) support services as a requisite of the funding. While such services (counseling, transportation, outreach) could represent important aspects of the physician's model of patient care, they spell economic losses for the practice.

In terms of prices charged, sponsorship can also create a special condition in which a sliding-fee schedule is required in order to ensure low-income residents accessibility to the practice. Sliding-fee schedules are financially draining because of high administrative costs and invariably require cross-subsidization of patients.

Finally, practices which are under public sponsorship usually reflect a contemporary emphasis on the primary-care medical model. This commitment to primary care may override economic pressures to achieve practice self-sufficiency (Feldman, Deitz, and Brooks 1978). Such an orientation away from lucrative, hospital-based medical care can compound other constraints on profit-making behavior applied by the outside sponsor.

Although the source of outside sponsorship varied, all the currently sponsored practices studied had a set of common organizational patterns.[2] These included salaries of physicians, a community board, and managerial oversight (or a salaried administrator).

Research Findings

If sponsorship of a practice means the need for special financial bolstering, then it follows that the sponsored practice's net income from operations does not parallel that of the similar private practice. Are high costs or low revenues to blame? In the last chapter it was shown that patient volume is the key to adequate revenues and low average costs for the practices studied. In comparing the revenues per physician of the unsponsored and sponsored physician practices (table 6-1), a difference of $26,500 was found. An even greater average difference in costs per physician—$29,500—was identified. The comparable figures for self-sufficient versus not self-sufficient were $34,000 and $24,000. (The income and expense differences between sponsored and unsponsored and self-sufficient and not self-sufficient are slight since the correspondence between self-sufficiency and unsponsored is so high. Only one of the non-self-sufficient practices was unsponsored.) The increased difference in costs suggests that the relationship of sponsorship to costs deserves close attention. These phenomena—lower revenues compounded by much higher costs—formed the basis for an analysis of the dynamics of sponsored-practice behavior. First, however, it was necessary to ascertain the importance of low prices and third-party reimbursement rates as an explanation for the subsidization of certain rural medical practices.

Are Lower Payments for Services the Main Problem?

One reason offered for the long-term financial dependency of many sponsored practices is the fact that they typically charge less. The phenomenon is attributed to the lower income level of patients served and to sliding-fee scales. Table 6-2 gives the average charges for each of the practices studied and illustrates the difference made when the average charge of the private practice is applied to the sponsored match. In most instances, there is an upward shift in practice net income, but only one sponsored practice would achieve self-sufficient status (physician net income in excess of $30,000) through such an adjustment. On an aggregated level, if the sponsored practices charged the same for office and hospital visits as their private counterparts, there would be an average increase in revenue per physician of approximately $10,000. It is apparent that only about one-third of the overall difference in revenues between the unsponsored and the sponsored practices can be attributed to prices charged. Offsetting any slight revenue increases would be the chronic problem of low volume. Moreover, high costs overwhelm any marginal increases in practice revenues for the sites studied. Collection rates do not vary that greatly for the sponsored- and private-practice pairs. These sponsored rural practices could benefit by the upward adjustment of prices and reimbursement rates. However, their ongoing dependence on external support results more directly from other problems.

Table 6-1
Per-Physician Practice Net Income for Fiscal Years Ending in 1978
(dollars)

Practice Description	Solo, Hospital in Town Unsponsored	Sponsored	Solo, 20+ Miles from Hospital Unsponsored	Sponsored	Group, Hospital in Town Unsponsored	Sponsored[a]	Group, 10 Miles from Hospital[a,b] Unsponsored	Sponsored	Extender Clinics[c] Unsponsored	Sponsored	Group with Two Satellites Sponsored
Revenues											
Ambulatory	48,089	29,127	41,110	70,524	47,790	42,450[a]	43,585	35,546	38,667	25,571	40,973
Ancillary	12,183	5,766	6,522	21,536	16,056	0	10,156	14,966	19,516	14,229	7,112
Nursing home	0	0	866	1,259	751	1,060	3,901	0	0	0	7
Hospital	37,335	22,627	9,444	0	56,761	7,197[a]	19,318	2,896	28,324	0	6,719
Total revenues	97,607	57,520	57,942	93,319	121,358	50,707	76,960	53,408	86,507	39,800	54,811
Expenses											
Medical											
Non physician salaries	11,150	24,647	11,426	8,075	10,266	4,576	15,671	20,953	55,386	25,064	24,026
Materials and fees	7,179	8,948	7,047	22,934	10,488	5,586	6,121	8,785	8,256	5,328	10,745
Administrative	16,545	31,589	17,911	23,954	25,126	15,738	7,199	29,630	27,592	12,698	37,909
Outreach	0	31,608	0	0	0	0	0	6,247	0	0	1,149
Plant	29,203	25,174	14,843	17,941	15,215	14,878	11,356	23,283	14,322	14,130	19,127
Total expenses	64,077	121,966	51,227	72,904	61,095	40,778	40,347	88,898	105,593	57,220	92,956
Per-physician practice net income	33,530	[64,446]	6,715	20,415	60,263	9,929	36,613	[35,490]	[19,086]	[17,420]	[38,145]

[a]Outpatient hospital revenue were included with ambulatory revenues by this practice.
[b]Year ending in 1977.
[c]Calculations for the extender clinics were made based on one full-time provider at each site, since the full-time-equivalent physician base is not appropriate.

Table 6-2
Potential Effect on Practice Revenues and Net Income of the Application of Unsponsored Charge per Encounter on Matched Sponsored Practice *(dollars)*

Practice	Average Charge per Encounter		Increase/(Decrease) in Total Revenues per Physician in Sponsored Practices with Unsponsored Average Charge	Resulting Practice Net Income per Physician
	Sponsored	Unsponsored		
Group 10 miles from hospital	15.05	11.98	(10,887)	(46,377)
Group with hospital in town[a]	14.10	18.55	16,050	25,979
Physician extender				
Group with hospital in town and two satellite clinics	14.76	18.55[a]	14,073	(24,072)
Solo with hospital in town	10.90	15.66	25,111	(39,335)
Solo 20 + miles from hospital	13.44	16.19	19,069	39,484

Note: The effect on practice revenues and net income was determined by using the actual collection rate of the sponsored practice. This table does not show the full effects of a change in service mix, which would be the probable cause of such a change in charge per encounter. Other factors such as changes in cost would result; however, their effect was not measurable.
[a]For purposes of comparison, the average charge per encounter of the unsponsored group practice was used as a "match" to the unpaired sponsored practice.

Dominant Behaviors Related to Sponsorship

The research results indicate that three dominant features characterize the behavior of sponsored practices. These practices tend to have lower physician productivity than their unsponsored counterparts. In addition, their administrative and facility (fixed) costs are disproportionately higher. Finally, they provide a mix of services which includes little or no hospital (inpatient) care.

Productivity: Physician and Plant Capacity

In their assessments of sponsored medical practices, federal programs have supplanted "self-sufficiency" measures with measures of productivity efficiency. However, the new emphasis on encounters per provider generally is not reflected in the behavior of the sponsored practices visited. For example, table 6-3 reveals a significant disparity between the number of encounters per

Table 6-3
Percentage Difference in Encounters per Physician by Matched Pairs

Practice	Total			Ambulatory		
	Unsponsored	Sponsored	Sponsored as a Percentage of Unsponsored-Practice Encounters	Unsponsored	Sponsored	Sponsored as a Percentage of Unsponsored-Practice Encounters
Group 10 miles from hospital	6,971	4,162	60	5,158	3,966	77
Group with hospital in town	7,919[a]	4,231	53	4,901	3,454	70
Physician extender clinic	NA[b]	NA	NA	NA	NA	NA
Group with Two satellite clinics/ hospital in town	7,919[a]	4,990[c]	63	4,901	4,248	87
Solo with hospital in town	7,581	7,158	94	5,193	5,469	105
Solo 20 + miles from hospital	3,814	7,620	200	3,207	7,530	235

[a]For purposes of illustrating differences, encounters for the unsponsored group with hospital in town are contrasted with the unmatched sponsored satellite with two clinics and hospital in town.
[b]Not applicable.
[c]Encounters of nurse practitioners and physician extenders are included.

physician for four of the matched pairs. For the fifth pair, the solo practice with a hospital in town, the difference is minor; other financial behaviors distinguish these practices. However, in the last instance, representing the extreme case for the unsponsored practices, the private solo practice 20 + miles from a hospital was languishing and, indeed, closed about one year after the site visit because of insufficient patient volume. The sponsored match, in contrast, resembles a private practice in behavior. It has an office patient volume comparable to that of any of the private sites visited. Interviews with this physician and financial records of the practice strongly suggested an imminent conversion to a nonsponsored, private practice. (More specifically, the physician had personally selected the site, an active practice from which a successful physician had just retired. He had then requested that the community request NHSC designation of the site, so that he could fulfill a two-year obligation.)

It could be argued that higher productivity per physician among the private practices results from the greater use of support staffing or greater proportion of hospital visits. When only ambulatory visits are included, the differences do narrow. However, sponsored practices which have lower productivity per physician also have more nonmedical personnel. They appear to be overstaffing, or staffing for peak-demand periods, and then bearing the costs of excess labor capacity when the volume of patient visits does not materialize. It should be noted that neither sponsored nor unsponsored practices adjust their staffing specifically to respond to fluctuations in patient volume.

The pattern of low productivity per physician prevailing in all but one of the sponsored practices is related not to the utilization of other medical personnel, but rather to the low volume of patients seen by the physicians. The low volume could result from the fact that the community's population has other sources of health care or that a salaried physician, who does not intend to remain in the community, has less incentive to dedicate himself or herself to building patient volume than does the private doctor who fully realizes that the "bottom line" is what remains after all other bills are paid. Or it could indicate that the delivery of good medical care at the practice translates into longer visits.

In this research, the physicians in the supported practices were not aggressive in attempting to change the practice volume. For instance, one group practice with low volume knew that a nearby busy private practice was closing, but made no attempt to work formally or informally to attract the retiring physician's patients. Although supported practices registered concern about the low levels of patient volume, the lack of practice-building activity can be interpreted as an effect of either the security of a guaranteed salary or the lack of a long-term commitment to remain in the area.

In contrast, many of the private practices exhibited strong practice-building patterns. The private physicians had become a part of the local health referral network. Even the physician who did not succeed in private practice, who had come to a locale where there had been no practice in five years, and who had distinct social and familial conflicts with the local community values still worked to gain entry into the referral network, aggressively seeking to build a specialization in home delivery to offset problems with low office volume.

Limits in their workspace or physical plant were not found to be constraining the productivity in sponsored practices. In fact, the findings on plant capacity clearly indicated a pattern of underutilized plant capacity in the sponsored practices. It has been shown elsewhere that there is a positive correlation of smaller facilities with success in achieving self-sufficiency (Feldman, Deitz, and Brooks 1978).

One example of the differences in excess capacity maintained in sponsored practices is depicted in table 6-4, which contrasts the number of encounters per examining room and the staffing patterns for the sponsored and unsponsored practices. On average, the sponsored practices conduct a strikingly lower number of examinations given the total number of available rooms.

Interpretation of the findings on plant capacity relates generally to the "grantsmanship" game which sponsored practices have to play. That is, they typically must develop proposals for funding to build or renovate which so impressively document the need for more space that the requested building may be far larger than current volume demands. They establish practices with forecasts of future volume in mind. Seeking grant support to build a medical facility is, most logically, a one-time endeavor. The excess capacity found in these practices may be utilized in the future. Practice behaviors, however, indicated a general lack of concern with defraying current costs, for example, through renting of extra space to private groups. It must be acknowledged that sponsorship creates a protective environment for practices, one on which the market does not impact too directly, and so practices may have no incentives to be incremental and conservative in expanding. Penalties are not levied, and indeed the costs incurred are often passed through to the outside sponsor.

Not surprisingly, the data on sponsored practices reveal that this pattern of operating with excess labor and plant capacity raises average costs above what they need to be.

Costs: Administrative Costs and Fixed Expenses

If we assume that their fixed costs are not extraordinary (for example, disproportionately high), unsponsored practices demonstrating higher

Table 6-4
Relationship of Total Office Encounters per Examination Room and Practice Staffing Patterns

Practice	Unsponsored (UN) Sponsored (S)	Total Office Encounters	Examination Rooms	Encounters per Examination Room	Staffing Patterns			
					Physicians	Medical Staff	Administrator	Nonmedical Staff
Group 10 miles from hospital	UN	12,483	3	4,161	2.4	3	0	2.5
	S	7,932	6	1,322	2	2	1	6
Group with hospital in town	UN	14,703	6	2,450	3	1.5	1	6
	S	6,907	3	2,302	2	1.5	0	3.2
Physician-extender clinic	UN	4,123	6	687	0.3	1 PA	0	2
	S	3,510	5	702	0.2	1 PA	0	2
Group with two satellite clinics and hospital in town	UN[a]	14,703	6	2,450	3	1.5	1	6
	S	12,744	14	910	3	0.5	1	8
Solo with hospital in town	UN	5,193	4	1,298	1	0	0	2
	S	5,469	4	1,367	1	2.5	1.5	4
Solo 20+ miles from hospital	UN	3,207	4	802	1	2	0	1
	S	7,530	3	2,510	1	1	0	2.3

PA = Physician assistant.
[a] For purposes of comparison only, the average chart per encounter of the unsponsored group practice was used as a "match" to the unpaired sponsored practice.

volume per physician are expected to show a lower per-unit cost. The cost differences combined with pricing policies determine the profitability of the practice.

The cost of providing care averages 50 percent higher for the sponsored practices. Table 6-5 breaks down the three cost elements used in the analysis of cost data. These differences in cost reflect the lower volume of the sponsored practices as well as the way in which the practice provides its services. If, for example, the sponsored group practice 10 miles from the hospital provided a similar number of encounters, its costs would have fallen from $21.36 to $12.75. If the outreach services had been dropped, the cost per encounter would have been $11.50, a cost which is way out of line with that of the private practices. This suggests that the practice is operating along a different production curve or has chosen a different mode of operation. Another way of expressing this is that increase in volume will not bring costs into line. This appears to be true with regard to administrative costs that are consistently high among the sponsored practices—on a per-encounter basis, 76 percent higher than for the nonsponsored practices.

The emphasis on the administrative model in sponsored practices creates a dramatic contrast with the group 10 miles from a hospital, the group with two satellites, and the solo practice with hospital in town. All three sites have a full-time administrator. In the sponsored group with hospital in town and the physician-extender clinics, both have hidden administrators; the group is managed, for a nominal fee, by the hospital administrator and controller, and the extender clinic receives extensive administrative directions from the staff of a state rural-health agency. If these costs were calculated in the practices' cost picture, they, too, would exhibit strikingly higher costs than their private counterparts. For the anomalous solo practices 20+ miles from a hospital site, the sponsored practice emulates the high volume and low administrative costs of the viable private practices, while the unsponsored practice's administrative costs are high because of its low volume. In fact, if its volume increased to that of the sponsored site, it is quite likely that its administrative costs per encounter would fall to about $2.50 or quite below that of the sponsored site.

Administrative Patterns

In this research, the general feeling was that the full-time administrator did not demonstrably affect the efficiency of the practice. The two practices with the lowest collection rates, for instance, have full-time administrators. In addition, the administrator's policy-making influence around issues of physician working hours, number of patient visits per hour, and physician availability for emergencies was minimal.

Table 6-5
Costs: Total Practice Cost (by Cost Center) per Encounter
(dollars)

Practice		Medical	Administrative	Outreach	Plant	Total
Group 10 miles from hospital	Unsponsored	3.13	1.04	0	1.62	5.79
	Sponsored	7.14	7.12	1.50	5.60	21.36
Group with hospital in town[a]	Unsponsored	2.63	3.18	0	1.90	7.71
	Sponsored	2.40	3.71	0	3.53	9.64
Physician extender	Unsponsored	13.83	5.99	0	3.13	22.95
	Sponsored	8.66	3.62	0	4.02	16.30
Group with hospital in town and two satellite clinics	Unsponsored	2.63	3.18	0	1.90	7.71
	Sponsored	6.96	7.59	0.23	3.85	18.63
Solo with hospital in town	Unsponsored	2.42	2.18	0	3.85	8.45
	Sponsored	4.69	4.41	4.42	3.52	17.04
Solo 20+ miles from hospital	Unsponsored	4.84	4.69	0	3.90	13.43
	Sponsored	4.06	3.15	0	2.36	9.57

[a]For purposes of comparison the unsponsored group with hospital in town was used to "watch" the sponsored practice.

Historically, a major emphasis has been placed on practice "administration" in the sponsored practices. In this research, with the exception of the physician-extender clinic and the solo practice 20 + miles from a hospital where the physician intends to convert to private practice, the outside sponsor has either mandated or financially encouraged the use of an administrator-clinician model. Contrastingly, for self-supporting practices, the clinician typically provides a substantial proportion of the managerial input, with office managers invariably responsible only for bookkeeping and carrying out policy decisions.

In sponsored practices, an administrator is often given a responsible role on the staff, although perhaps no true authority or control. Theoretically, to compensate for the difference in administrative costs she or he creates, the administrator must engender efficiencies in production and reduce costs or must increase revenues.

However, during site visits it was found that two key factors constrain the effectiveness of sponsored-practice administrators. First, the physician continues to retain all medical decision-making authority. Since medical decisions (for example, what is done to the patient, when and where the care is provided, and by whom it is provided) translate to practice-revenue policy, the administrator is virtually restricted to marginal impact activities such as improving collections or controlling plant costs.

Second, the administrator's time is frequently channeled into grant-generating or grant-management activities. Not surprisingly, the sites studied showed that administrators were most profitably spending their time soliciting grants. These grants could pay the administrator's salary, but simultaneously tended to increase the nonmedical (nonreimbursable) services which the practice was responsible for delivering to the community.

The implications of these constraints on administrators are clear when the effect of sponsorship is considered. Salaried physicians who share decision authority with an administrator are reluctant, in the practices observed, to implement changes which result in extra work, longer hours, and more time on the road between hospital and practice. They do not directly feel the financial consequences of their lower productivity. Ironically, the grant-hustling administrators observed were serving as another buffer for the physicians, further shielding them from the financial results of their low productivity by generating supplementary grant support to meet expenses.

Grant getting requires some ongoing administrative capacity, so the causality runs in both directions. That is, grant management often requires a full-time administrator or, at least, some additional administrative time and costs. Table 6-6 illustrates this relationship. The data show that the three sponsored practices with the highest administrative costs also have the highest level of subsidies per physician.

Table 6-6
Subsidy, Income, and Administrative Costs per Physician
(dollars)

Practice	Subsidy Income (Rank)	Administrative Costs (Rank)
Sponsored solo with hospital in town	106,194	29,627
Sponsored group 10 miles from hospital	78,719[b]	31,589
Sponsored group with satellites[a]	65,802	37,909
Sponsored solo 20+ miles from hospital	17,000	23,954
Sponsored group with hospital in town	16,500	15,736
Unsponsored group with hospital in town	0	25,125
Unsponsored solo 20+ miles from hospital	0	17,911
Unsponsored solo with hospital in town	0	16,545
Unsponsored group 10 miles from hospital	0	7,199

[a]In one instance, that of the sponsored group practice with two satellite clinics and a hospital in town, the scale of the practice and the potential for administrative efficiencies warranted the model. However, in that practice, the administrator did generate innumerable grants, but was quite constrained in his ability to affect the capacity-building behavior of staff physicians.

[b]Additional subsidies (relating to administrative services provided without charge) exist; however, these subsidies were not estimable.

A concern which emerges is that the practice development model requiring a full-time administrator may, particularly if applied to a small practice, set in motion forces which continually generate and renew grant support and, therefore, maintain the practice in a non-self-sufficient financial status.[3]

As a medical practice gets larger in terms of staff, patient volume, and number of physicians, the potential for a full-time administrator to generate savings from efficiency measures which go beyond the added salary costs increases. However, we found that the scale alone of the study practices did not justify an administrator-clinician model.[4]

Developing a network for health-care delivery, one which includes multiple sites, is clearly a task that demands administrator and clinician participation. However, for single-facility primary-care delivery, the scale that calls for the administrator has yet to be pinpointed by contemporary research.

Mix of Services: A Balance of Ambulatory
and Hospital Care

Patterns of service delivery magnify the behaviors of sponsored practices in regard to productivity and cost. Among these practices, including the exceptional solo practice 20+ miles from a hospital that is functioning in many regards like its private counterparts, the services mix does not reflect a balance of office and hospital inpatient care.

As seen in table 6-7, sponsored practices provide hospital care at a lower rate than their unsponsored counterparts. The data on individual practices in table 6-8 suggest that most sponsored practices are much less likely to hospitalize. The ratio of hospital to office encounters is three times greater for the unsponsored practices. The unsponsored practices have a ratio of 3.8 hospital encounters to 10 office encounters, while the sponsored have only 1.3 to every 10. The pattern of unsponsored practices corresponds to national averages; the unsponsored, therefore, are providing significantly less hospital care.

Because of variation in services mix, the sponsored practices show very different levels of hospital revenues. For the supported practices, only about 12 percent of their revenues derive from hospital-based services, as compared to an estimated 32 percent for the unsponsored practices. In terms of the net contribution, the difference is even more striking. For the sponsored practices, the net contribution averaged about $5,000 per physician, while it averaged approximately $27,000 per physician for the private practices.

These data suggest that the strong orientation toward the primary-care model among sponsored practices encourages behaviors which do not promote self-sufficiency. The question of whether hospitalization should provide the critical mainstay for rural medical practices is of utmost importance to federal policymakers. If they are to continue to provide grant support to practices on the basis of their being efficient, it will have to be argued that this support is preferable since it does not encourage expensive hospitalization. Clearly, the best use of the term *efficient* would be that the total health needs of the population served are being met at the least possible cost.

One could argue that the sponsored physicians on salary were providing care more efficiently by not encouraging excessive office visits or hospital admissions and, furthermore, that if the existing fee-for-service reimbursement system meant that insufficient revenues were earned, then special grants should be made. This logical argument hinges on the assumption that the sponsored practices are taking care of all the medical (or physician) demands of its patients. The orientation of the physicians towards primary

Table 6-7
Hospital Encounters per Physician and as a Percentage of Office Encounters

	Unsponsored	Sponsored
Average hospital encounters per physician	1,831	657
Hospital encounters per clinic or office encounter	0.38	0.13

Table 6-8
Hospital Revenues per Physician and as a Percentage of Total Revenues

Practice	Unsponsored		Sponsored	
	Hospital Revenues ($)	Percentage of Total Revenues	Hospital Revenues ($)	Percentage of Total Revenues
Group 10 miles from hospital	19,318	25.1	2,896	5.4
Group with hospital in town[a]	56,761	46.8	7,197[b]	14.2
Physician extender	28,324	32.7	0	0
Group with hospital in town and two satellite clinics	56,761[a]	46.8[a]	6,719	12.3
Solo with hospital in town	37,335	38.3	22,627	39.33
Solo 20+ miles from hospital	9,444	16.3	0	0

[a]For purposes of comparison.
[b]Does not include outpatient hospital revenues.

rather than comprehensive care and their isolation from other practitioners in the community suggest that the assumption would not hold up under examination.

What is the primary-care orientation that leads doctors away from the provision of hospital care? The public agencies and private foundations which typically fund rural medical practices strongly believe in preventive, ambulatory care. The physicians recruited tend to espouse these beliefs as well. Often, sponsored physicians are somewhat isolated from the mainstream of local medical care because, as they report, they are "stigmatized" as poverty-program doctors. The primary-care orientation of these physicians may actually be triggering the development of a dual health-care system. In this system, the sponsored family practitioners/primary-care physicians have a small and circumscribed delivery network, one which excludes specialty and hospital care. Meanwhile, their private-practice peers participate in the local networking of an entire range of referral, office, and hospital services. Unless the sponsored practices take responsibility or oversee the medical needs of their patients, the individuals who use them for primary care may utilize the private network for secondary and tertiary care. Higher costs and poorer quality would result from such a dual health-care system.

The different medical-care orientations of the sponsored practices, the lack of incentives on the part of sponsored physicians to develop a permanent practice, and public or community oversight of the sponsored practices all contribute to impede the interaction between private and sponsored-practice physicians. Since the demand for medical care of the newly established practices depends on this interaction—physician referrals or at least acceptance from existing practices—new sponsored practices are likely to suffer disproportionately in terms of the development of a patient following and the maintenance of the practices' patients.

The sponsored clinic with two satellites had two board-certified internists, who seek to follow patients in the hospital and who assist in surgery on their patients, and a physician who was chief resident of one of the small, outlying hospitals. However, the aversion of these physicians to what they termed *overhospitalizing* among their local peers had further removed them from the local referral network and isolated them in the primary-care mode. They saw no way that their commitment to preventive ambulatory care could be compatible with the provision of hospital care to a large number of patients.

In another example, of the group with a hospital in town, the attitude of the senior physician who strongly professed that their practice's lower hospitalization rate reflected the ability to care for patients on an ambulatory basis shows this firm primary-care commitment. For this practice, there was one hospital encounter for every twenty office encounters. This practitioner was convinced that on a per-capita basis the practice was saving the health system thousands of dollars. Health-expenditure data on the practice's patient population were not collected, so this observation cannot be addressed here. But because of the tradeoff between self-sufficiency and hospitalization, this is a most important issue that deserves the highest priority in future health-services research.

Illustrative of the premium placed on hospital care by some private practices was the action of the group with high hospital revenues; a newly recruited physician was asked to leave after a short period, because for most major problems he was referring patients to specialists in a nearby metropolitan area. The practice felt that their own practitioners were trained to provide most of the medical services needed by their patients.

Concluding Comments: Behaving as a Sponsored Practice

It may be argued that the behaviors which characterize sponsored practices are not *caused* by sponsorship per se. The fact that some practices grow out of sponsorship and become vital, viable parts of the private health-care network verifies that sponsorship does not prevent financial independence.

The findings discussed in this section suggest that it may be the *form* of sponsorship (for example, the imposition of the administrative model, a guaranteed income to a physician not intending to stay, the exclusive emphasis placed on primary-care services) which creates chronic dependence on outside support. Of course, the behaviors found among the sponsored practices are not restricted to supported practices. In the private sector, these behaviors would have to change, or else the rural practices could not survive. Unable to develop a patient following, the physician with low volume closed his doors shortly after this research was completed.

Administrative models of group practice where the physician is on salary have been quite successful. They have been able to keep costs down, maintain high productivity, and as a result have been financially successful. Rural areas, because of their size, may not lend themselves to such a model. The administrative model also works better when the patient volume is adequate. If, when the new practice was opened, the local residents all sought out the practice for care, the administrator would establish work and patient schedules. However, when the demand is not there, how is the administrator-clinician practice to encourage it? In newly developing health-maintenance organizations, a marketing staff is assigned the responsibility for seeking new patients. Neither the clinic administrator nor clinicians have that responsibility. In addition, the limited interaction between the clinicians in sponsored and private practices reduces the probability that private physicians will refer patients to sponsored practices.

Federal and other grant programs designed and developed on the basis of assuming severe access problems appear inadequately structured to build up patient volume. Understanding practice development is, therefore, crucial if we are to establish new medical practices throughout rural areas. This is the focus of the next chapter.

Notes

1. For the comparative analysis of unsponsored-sponsored practices, data from all eleven practices were included. These include five matched pairs of one sponsored practice which was not matched during the data-collection phase; for purposes of comparing practice functions and behavior, however, this practice is integrated into the analysis. (See chapter 2.)

2. Sponsored sites were financed by Rural Health Initiative grants, the NHSC, church funds, and a private foundation grant. It should be noted that all but the sponsored extender clinic were in designated HMSA service areas.

3. The definition of self-sufficiency used, since it excludes non-patient-generated revenue, does not incorporate the successful activities of the grants administrator. At health-care settings which conduct research and/or

educational activities, for example, a medical school, the successful activities of the grants administrator are included in the institution's revenues, and consequently the grants administrator is viewed as a necessity.

4. In one instance, that of the sponsored group practice with two satellite clinics and a hospital in town, the scale of the practice and the potential for administrative efficiencies warranted the model. In that practice the administrator did generate a number of grants, but was quite constrained in his ability to affect the capacity-building behavior of staff physicians.

7 Practice Development

This in-depth study of rural practices has found that practices dependent on outside financial support have fewer office visits and, even more important, fewer hospitalized patients. A conclusion from our field work is that the rural environment does not lend itself easily to new-practice development.[1] New medical practices strive to succeed in an environment composed of low population densities. Relatively quickly, a new practice needs to "convert" a high proportion of the population to use its services, both ambulatory and hospital. This may be unrealistic in areas where patients remain loyal to existing providers. Also, if the rural physician practices are too far from the hospital, she or he may refer patients to other physicians or the patients may have formed a patient-provider relationship with a physician close to the hospital. Further, few physicians are adequately prepared in skills of practice development to accomplish this task.

At the same time, the research has documented rural practices generating high patient volume and adequate physician net incomes. How does one explain these differences in practice development for areas where there is anticipated demand because of designated medical shortages?

The purpose of this chapter is to further examine the developmental process of rural practices. The discussion has two parts. First, we explore the elements of patient volume development and its two major components, penetration rate and use.[2] Penetration rate refers to the proportion of the community which uses the practice, while use refers to the proportion of total visits or care provided by the practices. It is important for the financial success of rural physicians to treat a high proportion of the community and to provide a high proportion of the services consumed by those who use the practice. Second, we discuss how the practice can affect these major components and why the physician, acting in an entrepreneurial role of practice building, is essential to the process.

Patient Volume

Our findings document that even for practices with high expectations of success, the development of office-based patient volume can be problematic. In table 7-1 several things are noteworthy. First, only one of the physicians had an office-based encounter rate approximating national

117

Table 7-1

Total Practice Encounters and Physician Primary-Care Encounters for Nine Rural Practices

Practice	Service-Area Population	Total Practice Encounters per Year[a]	Total Office-Based Encounters	Physician Office Encounters per Physician
Sponsored solo with hospital in town	10,000	7,158	5,469	4,310
Unsponsored solo with hospital in town	11,900	7,581	5,193	4,950
Sponsored solo 20+ miles from hospital	6,000	7,620	7,530	7,530
Unsponsored solo 20+ miles from hospital	5,000	3,814	3,207	2,909
Sponsored group with hospital in town	4,000	8,462	6,907	3,453[b]
Unsponsored group with hospital in town	8,063	23,757	14,703	4,284
Sponsored group about 10 miles from hospital	10,000	8,325[c]	7,932	3,966[d]
Unsponsored group about 10 miles from hospital	10,000	16,872	12,483	4,541
Sponsored group with two satellite clinics and hospital in town	26,000	14,972	12,744	3,017

[a]Year used for calculations was most recent twelve-month period for which data were available, usually 1978.

[b]Also includes inpatient hospital care.

[c]Excludes psychologist and dental encounters.

[d]Also includes physician-extender and nurse encounters.

norms for primary care reported by several research studies. Frequently, the office visit (encounter) rate was below even that of the 4,200 suggested for federally sponsored programs. The practice with the highest number of primary-care encounters per physician was one in which an energetic young physician, a native of the state, had taken over the practice of a long-established physician, inheriting a large office-based patient load, a physical facility, and a trained receptionist. Other new practices, even ones which had been established somewhat longer, found it difficult to generate this type of volume.

In the previous chapters on the determinants of self-sufficiency, it was pointed out that office volume may be less important than hospital encounters in terms of self-sufficiency. It should not be forgotten that the hospitalized patients of these rural practices are referred through the office. Thus, for general medical rural practices, an active office practice is necessary. One of the bases for both public and private sponsorship of medical practices is that they will become self-sufficient or develop an adequate patient following within a reasonable time. Typically, the NHSC physician has served for two years at one site. Rosenblatt and Moscovice (1978) suggest that this should be enough time for arriving at self-sufficiency if there are an adequate population base and other positive environmental factors, such as the presence of a hospital.

For the most part, the practices included in this research grew slowly over time, meaning that two years is a very brief period in which to generate an adequate patient volume. One surprising finding, shown in table 7-2, is the relatively small percentage of persons who remained active patients with some practices (had been to the practice within eighteen months prior to the patient-file survey). Some of the practices had retained as few as 50 percent

Table 7-2
Percentage of Patients with Initial Visits in Each Year

Practice	Percentage of Patients with Initial Visit						Percentage of Active Patients
	1973 or Earlier	1974	1975	1976	1977	1978	
Sponsored solo with hospital in town	7.5	7.6	16.8	17.8	25.4	24.9	61.8
Sponsored solo 20+ miles from hospital					45.2	54.8	100.0
Unsponsored solo 20+ miles from hospital					48.0	52.0	100.0
Sponsored group about 10 miles from hospital	2.5	4.1	13.1	26.2	20.5	33.6	81.1
Unsponsored group about 10 miles from hospital	13.9	21.8	16.7	18.3	16.9	12.3	57.8
Sponsored group with two satellite clinics and hospital in town				27.5	36.5	36.0	83.3

of those persons who had used the practice at least once. Others had been able to retain over 75 percent. Those practices with a lower retention rate either must be able to draw from a larger service-area population in order to ensure a steady stream of new patients or must see their existing patients more often. The high proportion of inactive patients suggests that many residents are interested in making contact with a new physician, but still desire to maintain their previous provider relationship.

Another way of examining practice growth is through a comparison of actual and expected growth patterns. Table 7-3 gives the results of providers' and administrators' responses to a structured question asking what had been the expectations for growth and whether the practice had actually fulfilled those expectations. There were as many practices which demonstrated a slower growth rate as there were practices growing as rapidly as anticipated. Few practices grew more rapidly than expected. Those practices with both high expectations and actual patterns of growth represented unique situations. The solo physicians more than 20 miles from a hospital took over an established practice upon the retirement of the resident physician. There were few alternative providers nearby. Clinic A of the group practices with satellites was the main clinic site established in response to local concern that other providers in town were so overloaded that they had closed their practices.

Ingredients of Patient Volume:
Penetration and Use

The two essential ingredients of patient volume are penetration[3] (the proportion of area residents who are active patients of a practice) and use (how many visits patients have with a particular physician per year). A high penetration rate indicates that there are few alternatives for medical care or that a particular provider is preferred.

Penetration Rate

One potential problem for a rural practice is that if the population base is relatively low, a physician must penetrate that market at a very high level in order to generate sufficient patients for self-sufficiency. Studies by Craige (1977) in Appalachia and by Kane, Dean, and Solomon (1978) in Utah indicate that even some practices penetrating over 50 percent may still fail to generate adequate revenues for financial self-sufficiency and continue to require support.

Craige suggests that physician practices could penetrate over 50 percent

Table 7-3
Physicians' and Administrators' Perceptions of Practice Growth

Practice	Perception of Practice Growth				
	A	B	C	D	E
Sponsored solo with hospital in town			X	X (Admin.)	
Unsponsored solo with hospital in town		X			
Sponsored solo 20+ miles from hospital	X				
Unsponsored solo 20+ miles from hospital				X	
Sponsored group with hospital in town	X	X			
Unsponsored group with hospital in town					X
Sponsored group about 10 miles from hospital		X		X	
Unsponsored group about 10 miles from hospital		X	X		
Sponsored group with two satellite clinics and hospital in town	X Clinic A	X Clinic B		X Clinic C	
Sponsored physician-extender clinic		X (Bus. Mgr.)		X	
Unsponsored physician-extender clinic				X	

Responses are from providers unless otherwise noted.
A: More rapid than anticipated and higher total patient volume.
B: As rapid as anticipated, with expected total patient volume.
C: Total volume anticipated, but more fluctuations in rate of growth expected.
D: Less rapid and with lower total volume than anticipated.
E: Other (less rapid but higher total volume—slow start).

of the service-area market within a relatively short time. Table 7-4 shows the penetration rates for the practices studied. Only two of the practices approached or exceeded a penetration rate of 50 percent. The practice with the highest penetration rate had been established the longest of the practices studied (nine years), had little competition from other providers except through relatively long travel distance, and offered a scope of medical ser-

Table 7-4
Penetration Rates for Seven Rural Practices

Practice	Service-Area Population[a]	Number of Patient Folders	Number of Active Patients	Penetration Rate (%)
Unsponsored solo with hospital in town	11,900	3,240	3,240	27.2
Sponsored solo with hospital in town	10,000	4,640	2,780	27.8
Sponsored solo 20 + miles from hospital	6,000	2,560	2,560	43.0
Unsponsored solo 20 + miles from hospital	5,000	1,510	1,510	30.0
Sponsored group about 10 miles from hospital	10,000	5,080	3,960	39.6
Unsponsored group about 10 miles from hospital	10,000	8,660	4,980	49.8
Unsponsored group with hospital in town	8,000	5,540	5,300	65.7
Sponsored group with two satellite clinics and hospital in town	26,000	4,262	4,080	15.7

[a]Service-area population was calculated from community statistics, where available, or from the provider's best estimate of the area served. These latter estimates yield less approximate estimates of penetration rates than do community surveys.

vices that would be the envy of most rural practices. Generally, the practices with the highest penetration rates were also the most self-sufficient. Of the three practices with penetration rates over 40 percent, two have been expanding self-sufficient practices for several years. The third is the sponsored practice with the very high patient volume which had taken over a long-established practice. By contrast, the unsponsored solo physician with a penetration rate of 30 percent has since left that community.

One of the reasons why sponsored programs have had such difficulty achieving a high patient volume is that they have often chosen to start new practices rather than enlarge those in existence. However, the predominant behavior for private physicians is to join an existing group. A new rural practice may require a major change in utilization patterns if the practice is to become self-sufficient. During several interviews in the course of the authors' research, physicians related the fact that no other physicians had come into the area except by joining an established practice. One implication of these findings is that, for a number of locating physicians, the problems of predicting penetration and utilization are eliminated by joining an established practice which provides a patient-volume base.

It is interesting to speculate what penetration rates a rural practice must achieve for financial stability, a subject not given much attention in the literature. One might hypothesize that it takes an active patient volume of 2,500 to support a primary-care physician at an income of $30,000.[4] Table 7-5 shows the penetration rates necessary to achieve this patient load in communities of different sizes.

It is readily apparent that a physician working in a very small service area of 2,500 must be able to achieve a penetration rate of 100 percent to generate a sufficient number of patients. In contrast, a provider in an area of 100,000 need only achieve a 2.5 percent penetration rate to have the same number of patients. It may be quite unrealistic in most small communities to expect a new provider to "sell" the new medical care to a large proportion of the community in a short time. The lower penetration rate needed for an adequate physician income helps to explain why doctors have established practices much more easily in urban areas and why even within rural areas there has been a concentration of physicians in more urbanized places (see Hassinger et al. 1975).

Moreover, a physician in a very small community must be able not only to achieve a high penetration rate, but also to retain these patients over time, and sometimes be in competitive situations with other providers who might move into the area. This helps explain the animosity occasionally expressed by the physicians already in established practices toward new sponsored physicians moving into a designated shortage area. In urban areas, each existing physician may lose a small proportion of patients to a new sponsored practice. Rural physicians, on the other hand, may be subject to substantial reductions from an additional practice and can identify the specific practice responsible. If the substantial increase in sponsored urban practices planned over the next few years actually occurs, one could expect

Table 7-5
Penetration Rates to Achieve an Active Patient Volume of 2,500 in Communities of Different Hypothetical Sizes

Community Size	Penetration Rate (%)	Active Patient Volume
2,500	100	2,500
5,000	50	2,500
10,000	25	2,500
25,000	10	2,500
100,000	2.5	2,500
1,000,000	0.25	2,500

to hear similar concerns raised by private practitioners in these communities as well.

Finally, the achievement of a high penetration rate may be a mixed blessing for a physician in a very small area. In this study, more than one provider spoke of the stress caused by knowing he was the only provider used by many people and "seeing your mistakes walk down the street every day."

Nevertheless, from the above discussion, it should be obvious that the accurate calculation of possible penetration rates is essential for predicting which rural medical practices will succeed. The smaller the service area, the more important it becomes.

Practice Use

The second element of patient volume is use—how many times per year a patient uses the practice and therefore what proportion of that person's total medical expenditures the practice is able to secure. A critical element to the survival of any practice is the way in which total utilization for a service area is divided among the practices serving that population. A comprehensive scope of services[5] allows a practice to address a wider range of problems and thus to increase its likelihood that use for that practice will approximate total physician-care utilization for the patients who use the practice. The earlier chapters highlighted the importance of providing hospital care for the patients served. The practice identified in this book as most financially successful has a large hospital patient volume, conducting medical as well as surgical procedures in the hospital. By providing a wider range of hospital services, it performed many of the lucrative procedures that its service-area population received. The physicians were aware of the importance of their providing the care to patients and not returning them to specialty physicians in the nearest city. In fact, when a young physician brought into the practice exhibited a much stronger preference for returning his patients to specialty practices, the physician was let go.

National data on physicians' incomes suggest that over half of their income is derived from hospital services. In our research on rural practices, the proportion coming from the hospital for the self-sufficient practices was higher. The ease with which the physicians can get to the hospital to serve the patients is significant. In the practices 20 or more miles from the hospital, solo physicians said that they would have to close down their office to provide the hospital care. One decided against it. The other physician closed his practice for 2 to 2½ hours in the middle of the day to drive to the hospital. Taking so much time away from the office may prove damaging in terms of building up patient volume. Yet, self-sufficiency for rural practices seems to depend on hospitalization. For the unsponsored practices, the physicians who were located closest to the hospital had the highest rates of hospitalization. It is unclear how much of the difference is explained by the greater proximity of the hospital and the physicians' style of medicine, which, in part, contributed to their locating varying distances from the hospital.

Hospitalization provides a physician with a greater share of the service area's physician expenditures. In 1976 the average person in the United States spent $551.50 for health care, $120.67 of which was for physician services (U.S. Dept. of Health, Education and Welfare 1978). By 1978, the year for which project financial data were collected, this physician expenditure was probably around $140. By offering a more comprehensive array of services, particularly hospital care, a physician retains a higher proportion of these health-care dollars. Fewer patients are referred for care, so more medical-care dollars are retained within the service area.

A hypothetical situation is illustrative of the impact of retaining a higher proportion of physician expenditures. For the sake of discussion, it was assumed that the revenue goal of each physician is $100,000 (this is the "ball-park" revenue level of the self-sufficient practices studied). Table 7-6 shows that 2,500 patients must spend $40 each to produce practice revenues of $100,000. If one postulates, for the sake of discussion, that the hypothetical service-area residents spend as much on physician's services as the national average, this practice is retaining only about one-third of physician-services expenditures. If, however, a practice is able to retain more than half the per-capita expenditure, or $100 per patient, a practice would need only 1,000 patients. Revenues per patient above $30 or $40 reflect a greater use of the hospital and the performance of expensive procedures, both in the office and at the hospital.

To provide the majority of physician services, a practice must perform both primary and secondary care. In urban areas, a large patient population

Table 7-6
Revenue per Patient and Population Necessary to Generate Practice Revenue of $100,000 per Physician

Population	Revenue per Patient ($)	Percentage of National-Average Expenditure	Practice Revenue per Physician ($)
2,500	40	29	100,000
1,333	75	54	100,000
1,000	100	71	100,000
800	125	89	100,000
715	140	100	100,000

may allow a primary-care practice to become self-sufficient, perhaps with little or no hospitalization. In rural areas, the smaller patient population means a primary-care-only practice with little or no hospitalization. This practice will have much greater difficulty becoming self-sufficient. Successful rural physicians must be able to perform a wide array of medical services and maintain their competence although they may have little actual experience performing some of the less frequent procedures.

Table 7-7 demonstrates that six of the practices studied recouped, on average, 25 percent of the national average of physician expenditure per person. With one exception, the average revenue per patient does not appear to exceed the ambulatory-care expenditures. This suggests that most rural physicians need to be the only physician for 2,500 people. Several explanations are possible for the low average expenditure: Per-person expenditures in rural areas for medical expenses are considerably lower than the national average, and even by recouping the entire amount, rural practices would still generate fewer dollars per person; patients of the studied practices divided their utilization among two or more practices and used the other practices more than those studied; or the practices studied generated a

Table 7-7
Revenues per Active Patient for Six Practices

Practice	Revenues per 18-Month Period ($)	Number of Active Patients	Revenues per Active Patient in 18 Months ($)	Revenues per Active Patient in 12 Months ($)
Sponsored solo physician 20 + miles from hospital	121,901	2,560	47.61	31.74
Unsponsored solo physician 20 + miles from hospital	78,362	1,510	51.90	34.59
Sponsored group 10 miles from hospital	145,571	3,960	36.76	24.51
Unsponsored group 10 miles from hospital	263,950	4,980	53.00	35.33
Unsponsored group with hospital in town	522,426	5,300	98.57	65.71
Sponsored group with satellite clinics	228,035	4,080	55.89	37.26
Average:			$48.96	$38.19

The methodology used above provides rough, "ball-park" figures since these are young practices and as they mature, the revenue per active patient probably increases. The 18-month figure divided by ⅔ thus probably yields a deflated estimate for the most recent year of practice.

relatively high number of encounters, but the patients used other physicians for hospitalization.

In the previous discussions on self-sufficiency and sponsorship, the orientation of sponsored practices toward primary care was discussed. The unsponsored practices appeared more interested and concerned about having an active hospital practice. The reasons are many. First, in general, physicians in the unsponsored practices had more residency training, making them better prepared to take care of patients in the hospital. These same physicians were also more cognizant of the alternative providers with whom they were in competition. Having a patient go elsewhere for more acute illnesses could mean losing the patient. Also, one can hypothesize some additional spillage effects. If sicker patients were sent to other physicians, then individuals might perceive the practice that did the referring to be less competent. There would be a tendency to go elsewhere for less critical illnesses. Thus, the lack of a hospital practice could reduce the demand for ambulatory care at the practice. Moreover, it seems reasonable to hypothesize that individuals would prefer a provider who can care for a wide range of their health needs. If the practice provides a wider scope of services, it allows patients to develop greater loyalty to the practice since they will not be coming into contact with other providers. This reasoning suggests that comprehensive providers should be able to secure a higher penetration rate, have less patient turnover, and generate more revenues per patient. Our data, unfortunately, are incomplete to test these hypotheses. However, the practice that provided the broadest array of ambulatory and hospital services did have the highest penetration rate, revenues per patient, and revenues per physician. Since hospital visits are more profitable, the net incomes of the physicians also were highest.

It is obviously easier for a physician with access to a hospital and office-based equipment for laboratory tests and procedures to retain a large proportion of physician expenditures and thereby become self-sufficient. Even if one had the dollars to invest in equipment, the risk inherent to the practice because of the need for a high penetration rate will mitigate against large, up-front expenditures by private physicians in rural communities. When a hospital is close, the risk is lower. However, because the availability and access problems are worse for isolated rural populations, there could be a tendency for the newest sponsored sites to be located farther away from the hospital. For these reasons, many new sponsored practices are not likely to be located in an environment conducive to self-sufficiency. The alternative to high revenues per patient is a large number of patients—again, *not* the environment of physicians practicing in sparsely populated rural areas. Because the existing reimbursement system virtually requires rural physicians to use the hospital if they are to become self-sufficient, newly established practices may be unable to survive without special assistance.

Such assistance may be warranted if the total cost of health care for the residents of the community is being held down substantially.

Alternative Sources of Care as an Explanation for New-Patient Volume

These findings suggest that the development of viable rural medical practices may be more difficult for all practices, sponsored or unsponsored, than previously anticipated. Even for "ideal" practices, those with high expectations of practice volume and located in designated medical-shortage areas, an adequate patient volume cannot be an assumed outcome for either sponsored or unsponsored practices.

Moreover, the data on practice growth indicate that practices generally did not acquire a majority of their clients during the first two years of operation. Practices with a longer operational history show a continued growth as well as an effort to replace patients who no longer come to the practice.

Why do persons in a designated shortage area fail to use a new provider? An explanation for this major anomaly suggested by our research is that practices vary in their ability to attract patients from a given population. Some of the reasons may involve lower utilization rates of certain rural populations. Some rural residents may use health care less often because they have lower expectations of the benefits of care.

Even more of the variation in use, however, may result from how the population's total demand for care is divided among the providers who potentially can serve a given population—the achievement of high penetration by a particular practice. The expected demand for care in a given population can be projected through community health planning. But it is difficult to explain why some providers have a heavy patient volume while others are operating below capacity, and why some populations prefer to seek care outside the community, leaving local doctors underutilized.

A key to understanding the dilemma of low penetration rates in designated shortage areas, found in conducting interviews for this research, was that the practices reported service-area residents generally had some source of medical care before the practices in our research were initiated, even if this care meant traveling long distances and inconvenient waits for appointments. Table 7-8 displays the providers' responses to the open-ended question: Where did people go for care before your practice was established? The verbalized answers can be grouped under the headings of other physicians and emergency-room services. Although there might be some persons in each of the service areas who had no care or inadequate care, not one of the physicians mentioned this spontaneously. A later ques-

Table 7-8
Previous Sources of Medical Care

Practice	Other Physician			Emergency Room	
	Same Town	Nearby Town	Large City	Same Town	Nearby Town
Sponsored solo with hospital in town	X		X		
Sponsored solo 20+ miles from hospital	X	X			X
Unsponsored solo 20+ miles from hospital		X			X
Sponsored group with hospital in town		X	X	X	
Unsponsored group with hospital in town		X	X		
Sponsored group about 10 miles from hospital	X			X	
Unsponsored group about 10 miles from hospital	X	X			X
Sponsored group with two satellite clinics and hospital in town	X	X			
Sponsored physician-extender clinic	X	X			
Unsponsored physician-extender clinic	X	X	X		X

tion concerned goals for the practices. Some physicians listed meeting health-care needs where no care existed as a goal for starting the practice. However, it is significant that the locating physicians saw their communities as already having some level of care.

This finding is corroborated by recent national survey data prepared by Aday, Anderson, and Fleming (1980). Table 7-9 indicates only 7 percent of farm populations and 10 percent of nonfarm populations had no regular source of medical care in 1976.

One might argue that while rural persons generally have a regular source of care, some segments within the rural population, especially low-income persons, do not have a source of care. The same data, when broken down by persons above and below the government's poverty level, indicate that the results are similar—only a small percentage of the rural population describes itself as having no regular source of care (see table 7-10). In fact, the lowest-income persons are sometimes less likely to describe themselves

Table 7-9
Access to Medical Care, 1976
(percent)

Type of Regular Care in 1976	Rural		Non-SMSA Urban	SMSA	
	Farm	Nonfarm		Central City	Other Urban
Particular M.D./D.O.	88	84	85	71	77
No particular M.D./D.O.	˙5	6	6	14	10
None	7	10	10	15	13

Source: Adapted from L. Aday, R. Anderson, and G.V. Fleming, *Health Care in the United States: Equitable for Whom?* (Beverly Hills, Calif.: Sage Publications 1980), table 2.1.

as having no source of care than are higher-income persons. These figures do not indicate whether the individuals are getting enough care or appropriate care. While it is undoubtedly true that some of these who have a source of care are being inadequately taken care of, it is not clear that the residents know that or would be willing to switch providers even if they were aware of it.

Other studies have corroborated the high proportion of rural residents with existing sources of care. In a 1967 survey of four Missouri communities by Hassinger et al. (1971), 86 percent of households surveyed had a family doctor whom they used regularly. Moreover, other studies also support the findings of this research that the possession of existing sources of care is a major explanation for patient use or nonuse of a new provider. In the study conducted by the GAO, for example, the possession of other sources of care was cited as the main determinant of low practice use among the NHSC practices studied.

The impact of these patient-provider use patterns on a particular practice is illustrated in a longitudinal study of a county in rural Utah by Kane, et al. (1978). In a repeat of a utilization study first conducted in 1971 to examine the effects of the construction of a new hospital and placement of three NHSC physicians who had replaced two retiring practitioners, Kane, et al. found the number of persons who had used the medical facilities in their county seat during the previous year increased by only 1 percentage point (65 to 66 percent). At the same time, the number of persons who bought nonmedical consumer goods in their county seat increased by 4 percent. Since the new providers were the only physicians in the county, at least some persons who were willing to buy consumer goods close to home were still willing to travel outside the county for medical care. The application of national utilization data to a specific rural population must take into account that patients have multiple sources of care and that a new provider is often breaking into an established medical market. (Of course, there are some rare instances of areas so sparsely populated and so poor that there is virtually no source of care within a reasonable travel distance. No information exists to identify how many shortage areas in the country fall into this category.)

Table 7-10
Rural Farm and Nonfarm Residents by Income and Source of Medical Care
(percent)

Type of Regular Care	Farm		Non-Farm	
	Non-BPL	*BPL*	*Non-BPL*	*BPL*
Particular M.D./D.O.	88.4	88.4	83.9	85.1
No particular M.D./D.O.	3.7	8.5	6.7	4.6
None	7.9	3.1	9.4	10.3

Source: Unpublished data, Center for Health Administration Studies, National Opinion Research Center Medical Access Study, 1976.

BPL = below poverty level.

D.O. = Doctor of osteopathy.

If one assumes every medical market is a competitive one, the problem for a new medical practice is how to attain a share of that market sufficient for financial survival. This involves not only attracting those persons with no source of care, but also, for a much larger number, convincing them to break established patterns of care and to try a new provider. Some research into the impact of patient loyalty on medical-care use already exists, but much more needs to be done to help identify those community or consumer characteristics which help explain use or nonuse in specific instances.

If the policy decision is made to continue sponsorship to improve access to care, the more helpful question to ask for a new practice is: What factors affect market potential? This research has begun to identify critical elements which affect patient receptivity to a new provider, such as population mobility and the death or retirement of a previous physician.

These factors do not supplant the importance of demographics—whether there is a sufficient base of population to support a practice or whether higher socioeconomic status is likely to affect a high total utilization. Rather, they modify and extend the analysis of demographics typically performed before sponsorship of a new practice is confirmed.

Some previous work supports the importance of the factors outlined above. An Opinion Research Corporation survey conducted for the American Academy of General Practice found that the most important reasons for doctor switching were the patients' change of residence, the doctor's death or retirement, or a referral (Cahal 1962). A common characteristic is that all these factors involve some catalytic circumstance which is likely to cause medical consumers to break established patterns of behavior.

Population Mobility

Population mobility seems to be an important intervening variable which affects use of a new provider in a community of a given population base. The literature (McKinlay 1975; Jones 1974) indicates that population mobility has two important consequences: It breaks the ties to a former medical provider, and it helps create a progressive atmosphere where new ideas and models of medical delivery are accepted.

The importance of population mobility in affecting market potential was suggested by two practices examined in our research. Both had been started by solo physicians in the last two years. Both physicians were dedicated to rural practice and hoped to remain in the communities permanently. One practice was generating a healthy patient volume; the other was not.

A key to understanding the differential development of these two practices lies in the fact that practice 1 had two major factors working in its behalf: The present practices were already full (defining the maximum share of the medical market they were willing to treat), and the type of industry brought in many more people who both were without established providers and could not get access to established practices. Practice 2 had neither of these positive characteristics. But more importantly, since there were no new people moving into the service areas, the physician had to try to compete directly for patients already attached to another provider. These practices were not full and were themselves trying to gain a larger share of the medical market.

It is interesting to note that health maintenance organizations (HMOs) have been more successful in penetrating the market in areas with high population growth and/or high population mobility. A recent study conducted for the Federal Trade Commission hypothesized that the high HMO rate of growth in California (where 19.8 percent of the state's insureds are HMO members and more than half of the nation's 6 million plus HMO members reside) was due to ". . . the state's growing population, which brings to California people who do not have their own doctors" (Goldberg and Greenberg 1977, p. 23).

One major difficulty is that rural underserved areas often have very little population mobility. In these situations, the establishment of new practices based on the realignment of patient use, or the growth of small practices, may be extremely difficult.

Change in Medical Trade Patterns due to Physician Death or Retirement

If the establishment of de novo practices is difficult in many rural areas because of low population mobility, one possible solution is building on practices that already exist. In our research physician death or retirement was found to be an important ingredient of patient switching in a number of practices. Two practices are particularly illustrative. Practice 1 was a situation wherein an NHSC physician took over a successful practice within days of the previous physician's retirement. The high use encountered from the start allowed the practice to become more than 90 percent self-sufficient within eighteen months.

The matching practice, practice 2, was started after five years without a physician in the community. In this period, consumers had established loyalties to physicians in three towns 20 or more miles away. The physician was faced with an additional interesting dilemma in his choice of a hospital. There were three hospitals, all about equally distant from the site in different towns and different directions. According to the physicians, patients in the community were using all three hospitals and the physician in the same area. The physician made his hospital choice based on the complement of services offered at the hospitals, but faced the increased difficulty of convincing the community population to end their ties to their existing physicians as well as hospital.

Breaking existing medical trade patterns proved very difficult. After three years, the physician relocated to a practice near a hospital.

A new issue raised in this experience was the loyalty of the population to a hospital. It was not unusual to find rural families who, generation after generation, have been born and have died in the same hospital. Faced with an inadequate supply of physician services, they may have looked to the hospital as a source of care when they believed they were seriously ill. One explanation of the wide variation in the ratio of hospital to total encounters was that some practices are adequate for "colds and sniffles," while other more serious problems require going to a hospital. This suggests the need for the practice to actively try to become the case manager, if not the deliverer of hospital care. The patient who is referred and not followed up could be lost to the physician who sees patients at the hospital.

Unpublished data from the 1977 Health Interview Survey help to explain why the time lapse between the death or retirement of a physician and the establishment of a new practice is so important. Table 7-11 shows the time of the most recent visit for persons who visit physicians. For about three-quarters of the population, this occurred less than one year ago. By using the results, it appears that over 85 percent of the population who utilize physicians will have made an alternative care decision within one year after their present physician retired or died. In five years, a mere 3 percent of the population will not have made an alternative care decision. While one visit may not mean that stable patient loyalties have been established, repeat visits might; and this pattern develops usually within two or three years.

An Entrepreneurial Approach to Practice Development

If practices are to be more successful in the competitive rural environment, certain questions must be answered: How does one identify areas of potential high penetration and thus adequate patient volume? What elements contrib-

Table 7-11
Most Recent Visit of Those Persons Who Visited a Physician, by
Geographic Region and Place of Residence
(percent)

Selected Characteristic	Time of Most Recent Visit to a Physician			
	Less than 1 Year Before	*1 Year Before*	*2-4 Years Before*	*5 or More Years Before*
Geographic region				
Northeast	75.6	11.5	8.8	3.3
North Central	75.2	11.1	9.6	3.2
South	74.3	11.9	9.9	3.4
West	75.9	10.2	9.5	3.3
Place of residence				
SMSA	75.9	11.1	8.9	3.2
Outside SMSA	73.5	11.8	10.1	3.7

Source: Selected unpublished data from 1977 Health Interview Survey, National Center for Health Statistics, Public Health Service.
We include persons receiving care at a private doctor's office, doctor's clinic, or group practice. Data are age-adjusted to the 1970 civilian noninstitutionalized population.

ute to patient identification and practice growth? What management decisions affect practice building, and who is appropriate to make those decisions?

Even though these questions could be answered by other parties (program developers and so on), the conventional wisdom among rural health professionals and providers emphasizes the catalytic role of the physician in promoting the success of the practice. In this respect, the physician is very much in the position of an entrepreneur, of understanding practice building as a marketing problem, and of capitalizing on the opportunities in the community and medical environments.

This has not been a focus of previous research, however. Most of the literature relating to the topic makes the assumption that a practice volume already exists and that the question for investigation is how much of the dynamic of the physician-patient relationship is controlled by the provider. Studies have examined the question of provider-induced demand for services and the control that the physician has over both the stimulation of "need" and the setting of price for services offered (Evans 1974; Sloane and Feldman 1978; Reinhardt 1978). However, if our contention that the new medical practices in rural areas are very difficult to start is correct, a more basic issue is how to get patients to utilize a new practice, for physician-induced demand cannot operate until after the patients come to the practice. In the next section we explore the questions outlined above and the ability of most physicians to deal with them.

Identification of Viable Areas for New Practices

Calculating practice volume and the time it will take to build a financially viable practice is essentially a process of estimating all the factors that determine use and penetration rates.

Our field of work indicates that physicians are relatively unskilled in asking questions which would allow them to assess the potential for penetration and use. Most had known where other providers in the area were located, whether the community was, in general terms, "progressive," and what other community resources existed (banks, retail stores, and so forth). In the main, however, they had not considered factors such as the strength of loyalty to other providers, whether the population was mobile and susceptible to a new provider, and what opportunities were afforded by the medical community for emergency-room coverage and referrals. Some of these issues later became acutely important for the providers as they realized the effect on their own practices. Moreover, both sponsored and private physicians often expressed the frustration that the promises of positive opportunities presented by community leaders did not always materialize. The "need" of the community was expressed through the filtering screen of community leaders who were interested in other issues as well (for example, the impact of locating a physician on community development). In retrospect, providers realized that a more important indicator of patient volume was the felt need of ordinary community residents who were often relatively content with their long-standing relations with other providers.

Contributors to Patient Identification
and Practice Growth

Two factors in the medical environment (use of the emergency room and referral systems) are mechanisms by which new physicians can identify potential patients. The emergency-room services and referral patterns help put a new physician in contact with patients. Still, the practice must also have something to offer patients in order to cause them to switch from their present provider.

The development of referral patterns outside the practice seemed to be a function of interpersonal skills as much as of the surrounding medical community's tradition of cooperation or competition. Some providers expressed the feeling that some specialists were known to be "patient stealers" and tried to avoid referring patients to them. But generally physicians who were able to manipulate the referral systems to their benefit were also able to manipulate other parts of the medical environments as well as generate confidence on the part of their colleagues.

Referrals from one practice to another often increase the demand for care. If physicians complement rather than substitute for one another, they may all benefit financially from referrals, and the quality of care provided to their patients may be enhanced. If most rural as well as urban residents have existing sources of medical care, how do new practices develop an adequate patient following?

In addition to patients voluntarily switching from one practice to another, it would appear that physician referrals have to be significant. A significant number of referrals to a new practice could occur if the existing physicians wanted to reduce their patient load or if the new physician added a dimension of care that existing providers could not supply. In the former case, physicians would refer to new practices that are substitutes for them. Patients would switch practices. In the second instance, the referring practice would retain the patient, but some of the medical care would be delivered elsewhere.

A new practice must discover how it fits into the existing medical-care network, and then it must develop the referral patterns that will assist its growth. If referrals have to be significant and sponsored practices do not fit into the prevailing private delivery system, then sponsored physicians will have a much harder time identifying and securing new patients.

Most physicians saw the emergency room (ER) as a mixed blessing. It helped to identify patients, but it also consumed their precious personal time. Rather than using the ER as a marketing mechanism, most physicians saw it as an evil from which to escape as soon as possible. Some providers also felt a good deal of conflict over seeing another physician's patients, especially if the patients had not been receiving satisfactory care. The rediagnosis and represcribing of care could create personal and political problems within the community and hospital. Only one physician who was denied emergency-room privileges by the existence of an ER corporation articulated clearly the negative impact of this on his practice's development.

Process of Practice Building

Medical services are the commodity sold by a practice. Medical providers are central to practice operations. Their decisions fall across a wide spectrum—not only the content of the medical policies, but also the management of staff and a myriad of other issues for which clinical training has generally left them unprepared. Moreover, both the personal philosophy of the provider and the administrative structure of the practice may diminish the incentives for a physician to become involved in all the decision-making roles. The divisions of responsibility must be clearly articulated, and the provider who is not financially at risk must be motivated. One of the non-self-sufficient practices, managed by an administrative group, had not come to an agreement with one of their NHSC physicians. The physician had placed restrictions on his patient load which made efficient management of the practice exceptionally difficult.

To residents in a small community, the physician *is* the medical practice, and the popularity of the provider and the practice are intertwined. Further, if one assumes that the medical market is competitive for patients, then the physician who has direct patient contact must be involved with promoting opportunities to identify and attract new patients. Thus, the activities of a physician determine who comes into the practice. And his medical training and treatment patterns determine what happens to those who come into the practice. Thus, rural physicians find themselves engaged in all aspects of the business—sales, production, distribution, and financing.

Most of these physicians felt ill prepared by their previous training to make the variety of practice decisions required. Some had developed informal networks of communication to medical graduates a few more years advanced and used these networks for decisions about location, the purchase of equipment and other capital items, or whether to join a group practice or start out solo. Others had tried to supplement their lack of management knowledge by reading trade journals, attending conferences and workshops, and so on. In some cases this proved unsatisfactory because the input of knowledge came after crucial decisions had been made. Still others were dependent on a staff person such as a bookkeeper or an accountant to raise issues and supply the information on which decisions needed to be made.

The providers' interest in an entrepreneurial role relates in part to their personal philosophy about how medical care should be delivered. Some defined the role of the physician in clinical terms—one should not divert attention from the direct delivery of care to issues which should be handled by someone trained to do so. Others expressed a feeling that medical care in underserved rural areas should be permanently subsidized, and thus management and organizational issues were of secondary importance to issues of care delivery. Still others expressed feelings that medical services were less important than broader health services (health counseling, nutrition education, and so on) and that the provider's time was better spent orchestrating a comprehensive response to patients' range of health needs than concentrating on management or financial or reimbursement issues.

Finally, the organizational structure of the practice sometimes prevented a physician from being directly involved in management decision making. In the sponsored practices, the decision-making role was shared with an administrator, a different relationship from that with a bookkeeper or an accountant, who basically prepared information for the physician's decisions in private practices.

In sponsored practice, some providers were quite motivated to become central to practice-building issues and sought opportunities to become more knowledgeable and involved. Our sample of practices is too small to be more than suggestive, but the desire to be a focal decisionmaker seemed to be related to the provider's desire to remain permanently in the community.

The ultimate question is, of course, why some physicians function more in the role of entrepreneur than others and seem much more able to understand and engage in the process of practice development. Is it that some individuals are just more entrepreneurial than others and would be able to maximize their environments wherever they are? Are there personal philosophies of medical practice which preclude a physician from considering an entrepreneurial role appropriate? Are there critical pieces of management or marketing training that would supplement a clinician's ability to ask the relevant questions about practice location and engage in the process of practice development? What kinds of technical assistance could be provided to support practitioners with specific problems? Are there elements in the sponsored-practice system which, by removing the personal financial risk to the provider, remove some of the incentive for practice development? We suggest that all the above may be factors and are important topics for future research.

Concluding Thoughts

Our description of rural practices in 1978 having to compete for patients may seem at odds with other descriptions of rural areas suffering from severe medical-personnel problems. Obviously some areas have few, if any, physicians. Some residents will begin using a new practice the day it opens its doors. But most residents have located and are using other practitioners. If the new practice, sponsored or unsponsored, is going to have full patient complements, it has to attract patients away from their existing providers or have patients referred for some portion of their care. The existence of the practice with its closer proximity to the patients may be all that is needed. More likely, the entrepreneur of the practice, whether the administrator, community board, or physicians, must develop a strategy for practice growth. This is more likely to occur if the entrepreneur's well-being is dependent on the success of the practice and when the practice integrates itself into the prevailing medical-care delivery system.

Previous programs had a different perspective of the rural-health market. They were designed to put in place a practice, hospital, or physician to meet the excess health demand in the community. In short, the necessary demand was assumed to be there, and the newly placed practices just had to serve it.

Many of the individual sites failed, and programs have been continually modified. Some success stories exist. (The reader is reminded that all the self-sufficient rural practices we studied initially were given some support.) We believe that many of the failures can be tied to inadequate patient volume. The expected number of patients did not come through the doors, and when they did, the practices did not provide an adequate range of services.

The view of rural health care we have acquired over the course of the research—that of alternative sites competing for patients—suggests that new rural-health initiatives must incorporate the desire and means to compete with or complement existing practices as well as the incentives for success or penalties for failure. The organizational form of the entities as well as the financial incentives need to be considered in light of current reimbursement rates that encourage hospitalization and the location of practices in more populated areas and near a hospital. To encourage self-sufficiency under these reimbursement incentives may not yield the most efficient delivery system for the community. In the next chapter we consider some of the options for developing more responsive and socially desired practices.

Notes

1. A study conducted simultaneously for practices established in urban areas revealed similar major findings—inadequate demand and lower average revenues for the practices of federally sponsored programs. See Charles Brecher and Maury Forman, *Financing Urban Ambulatory Care Programs*, Washington, D.C.: United States Conference of Mayors, April 1980.

2. For this discussion, a distinction is made among the concepts of utilization, use, and penetration rates. *Utilization rate* is the total number of patient visits per person, per year:

$$UT = \frac{\text{total visits} \times \text{patients}}{\text{year}}$$

Use is the rate of visits to a particular practice i:

$$US_i = \frac{(\text{total visits}_i \times \text{patients}_i)/\text{year}}{(\text{total visits} \times \text{patients})/\text{year}}$$

Penetration rate is the proportion of persons in a service area who come to practice i, usually expressed in a reasonable "active patient" time frame of 18 to 24 months:

$$PN_i = \frac{\text{patients}_i}{\text{patients}}$$

3. Penetration rate is determined by the proportion of active patients per service-area population. For our research, active patients were defined

as those using the practice within the previous eighteen months. Other authors (for example, Craige 1977) have defined active patients as those using the practice within twenty-four months and have consequently calculated higher penetration rates. The method used to calculate penetration rates (the number of persons in the service area with active patient status) would tend to yield a lower ratio than would community surveys in which persons were asked to name their doctor. That is, persons could think of a doctor as "their" doctor even though they had not used the practice within the last eighteen months.

4. For this discussion we have assumed round numbers of 2,500 patients × 2 visits/year × $15/visit = $75,000 with a physician income of 40 percent = $30,000.

5. Laboratory, x-ray, hospitalization, surgery, etc. This argument assumes that the services are priced so as to be profit centers. As identified earlier, ancillary services often were priced by the practices so low as to be loss centers. If this is the case, the extent to which the practice increases the comprehensiveness of services could detract from financial viability.

Major Conclusions and Policy Choices

This chapter considers the major policy choices that evolve from our research on the final behavior of rural medical practices. In the discussion that follows, we first describe the ways in which rural medical practice can become more financially attractive to medical providers. We then summarize the organizational and structural changes that could be adopted for sponsored practices to make them more efficient and, therefore, more likely to become self-sufficient at some future time.[1] Our premise for these recommendations and focus is that while health-care policy cannot change the cultural amenities of rural areas, it can influence dramatically the financial well-being of rural practices.

Making Rural Practices Financially More Attractive

Because we analyzed only eleven rural practices in depth, the issues and problems discussed may not pertain to all newly begun rural practices. There is good reason to suppose, however, that the three key findings with regard to the financial well-being of rural practices will hold up to further study and that policy alternatives should, therefore, be considered at this time.

The three findings are:

1. Low practice volume is the major obstacle preventing self-sufficiency and one that newly established rural medical practices will encounter on their paths to self-sufficiency.
2. Reimbursement differentials between rural and urban areas in some states substantially reduce rural medical practice revenues.
3. A contemporary rural practice must hospitalize if the physicians are to earn incomes approaching the national average.

Starting a rural practice is financially less attractive than an urban practice to private physicians. Sparse populations usually mean that it takes longer for a rural practice to achieve a satisfactory level of patient volume. The impact of this longer development time is significant. Even if physicians were equally positive about living in a rural or an urban area and could earn the same real income with full practices, they would tend to con-centrate in larger communities because the shorter development time translates into greater lifetime earnings. As a result of lower third-party reim-bursement, rural physicians with a full practice may still have a harder time earning comparable incomes. Finally, the importance of hospitalization to a private rural practice may exceed that of urban practices since rural physi-cians have a smaller population from which to earn their incomes. Yet, the distance physicians have to travel between office and hospital may make hospitalization a risky venture, particularly for a practice trying to build up a patient following. Below, we analyze the development issues generated by low volume, the potential changes in reimbursement policies, and the system modifications that reduce the pressures on rural practices to hospitalize.

Developing Rural Practices:
Problem of Low Volume

In chapter 5 we showed that differences in the quantity of services provided per physician explain about 80 percent of the revenue difference between self-sufficient and non-self-sufficient practices. For the rural practices studied, it was found that physicians in 1978 could earn about $40,000 to $45,000 net income annually if they made 4,000 to 5,000 office visits and 2,000 hospital visits annually. To achieve this level of encounters per physi-cian requires high market penetration and use rates in sparsely populated rural areas. If no other providers are serving a rural, medically underserved community, then high rates may be possible to achieve in a short time.

For the practices analyzed, we found that the development of an ade-quate patient demand usually took years. An important reason for the inade-quate level of patient demand facing a new practice appears to be that most residents of a rural area presently have a source of care. The existing source of care might be over 30 miles away and may be used less than optimally. If, however, this source of care has been used for some time, it may not be displaced readily, even when a practice closer to the resident is established. The sparsity of the population in rural areas, plus the existing loyalty that in-dividuals feel toward their physicians, make practice-site selection and development of critical importance. Establishing a new rural practice appears to be a risky financial venture in the best of circumstances. Therefore, it is understandable why all the sites visited received some development support. Without special support for developing new rural practices, physicians are likely to start new practices in more densely populated areas and to join ex-isting practices, thereby further widening the physician/population ratio be-tween rural and urban areas. Thus a case can be made for special assistance to physicians willing to establish a practice in a rural community.

The type and length of special development support provided to the new rural practice, however, should vary with the desired goals. If, on one hand, the goal is to ensure that rural residents have health-care services available, then the strategy should be to put a practice in place and then let the interplay of the market forces determine whether adequate demand exists for a financially self-sufficient practice. If rural residents still travel great distances to their old source of care or for other reasons do not use the practice, then the practice would not reach maturity.

On the other hand, where the goal is to equalize the availability of physicians' services to rural and urban residents, then the first strategy of merely placing practices in rural areas will fall short of the goal. Because of the need to have a high market penetration rate, it probably will take more time for the rural physician, as compared to his urban counterpart, to develop a mature practice. A number of factors determine the length of time required to develop a practice: the number of residents looking for a new medical practice, the number of providers seeking new patients, and the number of contacts between the two groups. Our findings suggest that it takes years to start a new rural practice. By contrast, surveys done by *Medical Economics* suggest that new urban practices can be self-supporting in less than one year.

The longer it takes to develop a rural practice, the higher the likelihood of failing to reach practice maturity. This may be due to the unwillingness or inability of physicians to endure prolonged periods of low incomes. Moreover, a mature practice is able to bear higher levels of patient dissatisfaction and turnover. In contrast, a practice struggling to build a full patient complement risks a general loss of community acceptance with a few dissatisfied patients.

Policy Choices for Developing New Rural Practices

Getting Practices Started

With the goal of just ensuring availability of health care services to rural residents, the program objective is to find the most efficient way of starting practices. Small start-up grants combined with more information might be enough to attract physicians. The start-up grants could be for the renovation of space and purchase of equipment. Such support could come from the federal government, but participation from local residents may be an indicator and a predictor of local demand. The Office of Rural Health Systems in North Carolina uses such a strategy. By gathering information about the likelihood of a high level of demand prior to making the initial investment, the development funds could be spent in a more cost-effective way. Currently, the federal government spends a meager sum in designating a site as a medically underserved area as compared with the funding of the new practice. A greater effort in site selection may reduce the expenditure per site developed or maintained.

The current process of identifying a community as a health manpower shortage area largely depends on its physician/population ratio, although other social- and health-status indicators are included. The ratio does not assess the level of unmet demand or even unmet needs. A first step in acquiring such estimates would be to gauge the current utilization rates. Since individuals travel to see a physician, the lack of a physician in a community may not mean that the population is receiving no service or is being underserved. This information can be gathered by using survey research methods. A sample of the population in the community could be interviewed either in person or through the mail. The Office of Rural Health Systems in North Carolina has found in their surveys the most important question to be whether an individual currently has a regular physician or other source of medical care.[2] The utilization data could be used in conjunction with other measures to designate a location as being underserved or as a way of prioritizing the sites to receive investment awards. While there is no precise technique available to translate the utilization information into a probabilistic statement of success and although its usefulness should be studied further, it would seem to provide a better indicator than any we have now.

Other research should be conducted to isolate the factors that predict which practices are most likely to succeed. For example, a statistical analysis could be performed to ascertain the relationship between the practice volume of newly established sites and a number of socioeconomic and medical chacteristics of the area. Of particular interest would be the impact of the size, age structure, and density of the community's population; the prevailing population trends (growth, decrease, or turnover); and the number of providers within 10, 20, and 50 miles.

Start-up Plus Developmental Support

If the goal is to make physicians equally available to rural and urban residents, then physicians would have to become indifferent to starting a practice in an urban or a rural area. In terms of economic assistance during development, this would mean some start-up assistance, as well as longer-term operational support while the practice is maturing. The operating support would be compensating physicians for the income lost because of the longer practice-development time in sparsely populated areas. When the decision to provide developmental support is forthcoming, there still must be clarification of the duration, the amount, and of the type of support.

The start-up grant could be for a mixed number of years and at the same level of support for all practices. Or, it could vary in terms of both time and money according to the particular needs of the community. The view that practices require an incentive to compete for patients guided our thinking on the programmatic features.

How Long Is Support Needed? The duration of the grant could vary with the penetration rate necessary to have a specified active patient load. For illustrative purposes we use 2,500 per physician. Since one would want to assume some existing medical shortage, it seems reasonable to hypothesize that a new rural practice will be able to achieve some "target" penetration rate by the end of year 1, 2,. . . . Again, for illustration purposes only, a "target" rate of 25 percent for year 1 and higher rates for subsequent years are assumed. For example, if the expected penetration rates by year were

Beginning of year	1	2	3	4	5	6	7
Penetration rate	0	25	40	55	70	85	100

one would support practices starting up in smaller population areas for a greater number of years. With the patient target of 2,500, a practice in a community of 10,000 would receive support for 2 years while one with a population of 4,000 would be supported for five years.

How Much Is Needed? The level of support provided per physician could be the difference, or some part of it, between the total revenue that a rural practice would generate when fully developed and the level of revenue expected from a practice developing at the desired rate. To calculate the support level, the target revenue per physician would have to be decided. The target revenue for a mature practice would be determined by the expected patient load and per-patient physician expenditure for each of the development years. For illustrative purposes, once again, this might be $80,000 for a solo-physician rural practice. If, for example, the community has 4,000 people and the first-year penetration rate were 25 percent, the expected patient load would be 1,000 at the end of year 1. If each patient were assumed to spend $35 annually, the total expected revenue (the target) in year 2 would be $35,000 at a minimum. These figures would yield a potential grant of $45,000 in year 2 ($80,000 less $35,000). By using the growth in penetration rates set out above, the grant could be $29,000 in year 3 and $3,000 in year 4. If the actual revenues exceeded the target level, the amount of the subsidy would be reduced. This could be a dollar-for-dollar reduction or could be less to encourage practice buildup.

The expected revenue per patient could be varied to reflect the scope of service that should be delivered. Practices which would be expected to do more hospitalization would be assigned a higher expected per-capita revenue. If, in the above example, the expected per-capita annual revenue were $75, then the amount of the award in year 2 would be quite small and there would be no grant in year 3. By varying the expected per-patient revenue, the intended medical orientation of the practice could be incorporated. If, for example, the practice were far from a hospital or specialists were readily available, the expected revenue per patient would be lower. Such an adjustment allows a purely ambulatory practice to exist and does not create additional financial incentive for the providers to hospitalize at an excessive rate.

What Type of Support? In the above example, the grant took the form of a "last-dollar" revenue subsidy. The subsidy in this case could be used to pay practice costs or to provide the physician's income. One alternative would be to guarantee a physician or other medical workers specific incomes (a "first-dollar" subsidy). From a physician's perspective this might be more attractive since there would be no uncertainty about his/her income. From a programmatic perspective, it seems less efficient since the amount of subsidy varies inversely with the penetration rate and directly with practice costs. If the physician were guaranteed $30,000 annually and the net income from operations were only $1,000, the federal support for the physician's income would be $29,000. If the practice held its costs down or increased its patient load so that the net income from operations (income available for the physicians) was $25,000, the federal subsidy would be only $5,000. Under the current NHSC program which guarantees the salaries, such perverse subsidies exist. A "last-dollar" revenue-subsidy approach would encourage the practice to be more efficiently organized. Having too many nurses and aides or other excessive expenses would reduce the net income available to the practitioner for any given revenue.

Physicians have some influence over costs and collections, but more importantly over revenues because of their influence on patient volume and service mix. By setting a revenue target and subsidizing the expected deficiencies rather than providing a guaranteed salary, incentives for physicians to hold down costs and build up a patient following are created.

Rural-Urban Reimbursement Differences

Rural physicians will generate lower revenues than their urban counterparts with similar patient loads if they are reimbursed at a lower rate. In three of the six states visited, a differential urban-rural reimbursement-rate structure existed under Medicare. If we assume that difference extended to all payors, the rural physician in the Southern state would generate 20 percent less in total revenues, and the physician in the Midwest state would earn 8 percent less.

Reimbursement rates usually are established by the prevailing charge in the community. Since no attempt was made to explain the differences in charges in terms of costs, it is not clear whether the lower revenues translate to lower physician incomes. While rent and labor costs may be lower in rural areas, countervailing pressures may make rural practices more expensive. As small practices, they may not be able to benefit from economics of scale. Also, the day-to-day fluctuations of patient loads in rural areas could create pressures for more excess capacity in rural areas and, therefore, could mean higher fixed costs per encounter.

One explanation for the lower average charge in rural areas is that these areas have had a slower growth rate in the number of physicians. As new physicians enter a community, they are likely to set their charges at or near the upper end of those of physicians in the community. This pricing behavior is a response to third-party reimbursement policies, which often pay the physician whatever amount is lower—his own fee or some average of all fees in the community. By pricing at the upper end of the range of community charges, a physician will be reimbursed at the highest rate possible. As a result of this pricing behavior of the newest practices, the third-party reimbursement rates will be pushed up. This means that areas with a higher growth rate in physicians are likely to experience faster increases in third-party reimbursement rates. This scenario of how reimbursement rates are established and increased suggests that these ratios do not provide clear signals as to where resources (in this case, physicians) should move. In fact, the need for physicians and the level of reimbursement rates could be inversely related.

Because reimbursement rates do not necessarily reflect market forces, they should not be signals to physicians to locate in urban rather than rural areas. A statewide reimbursement rate could be established to equalize rates paid in rural and urban areas. Alternatively, a "rural-area premium" could be developed. The premium could be adjusted according to population density, estimated patient demand, and the service mix of the practice. For example, if a rural practice had little or no hospitalization, its average charge would be lower than practices that hospitalized. This could be adjusted for by allowing a higher premium.

Capture of Hospital-Based Physician Expenditures

On a per-hour basis, it is much more lucrative for a physician to see a patient in a hospital since rates for hospital care are higher than for an office visit. (This assumes that the length of time spent by the physician in conducting a hospital visit and an office visit are roughly equal.) In sparsely populated rural areas, a hospital practice may be even more important, since the number of office visits may be insufficient to yield a net income sufficient to keep the physician in the community. If the practice does not hospitalize, the number of active patients from a given population must be higher, or else the practice must see each patient a greater number of times during the year. This suggests that rural practices providing only primary care be given a longer period of start-up support in order to have time to secure the higher penetration rate. One problem with this solution is that a high percentage of the population may not want to go to a practice when it does not provide hospital care or may not come into contact with such a practice when in need of medical attention.

The rural practice placed in the greatest financial bind under the existing reimbursement system is the one a considerable distance from a hospital. A physician who must drive 30 minutes or more to the hospital may actually lose money when hospitalizing at a moderate rate. Only by hospitalizing a high percentage of the patients does it become financially beneficial for the practice. This has the obvious disadvantages of encouraging excess hospitalization and thereby increasing the cost of medical services for the entire population.

The economic incentives to hospitalize are faced by urban and rural physicians. Certainly efforts must continue at the national level to develop a reimbursement-rate structure which eliminates this incentive to use highly expensive resources. We hope our findings will contribute to the case for making such changes. Self-sufficiency which comes at the cost of unnecessary hospitalization is an inefficient use of society's resources. We do not know whether unnecessary hospitalization was occurring in the self-sufficient practices studied. However, the rate of hospitalization and the ratio of hospital to total encounters found in the practice with the highest physician net incomes were high in comparison to national norms. This finding raises the issue of whether the price being paid for self-sufficient rural practices exceeds the costs of subsidizing non-self-sufficient practices which hospitalize at a low rate.

If the rates being paid to physicians for ambulatory and hospital care were better reflections of competitive market forces, then the efficiency and self-sufficiency outcomes for practices would not be in potential conflict. That is, the most efficient practice (in terms of the delivery of health services for its patients) can be unprofitable because it does not provide unnecessary, but lucrative, hospital services. Because the necessary changes in the rate structure to remove this inconsistency are not imminent, alternative solutions for rural health-care practices must be developed.

One such alternative would be to have the revenues of rural physicians reflect the hospital expenditures of their patients, whether or not they provide the care. Preferably, this should be done so that total resources devoted to hospital care are not increased. This might happen when the rural practice is incorporated into a system that provides secondary and tertiary medical care. Making rural primary-care practices part of an organized, financially interrelated system of comprehensive care can be done in a number of ways. It would occur if spatially dispersed groups or partnerships were established. Alternatively, hospitals or HMOs could employ rural physicians or guarantee their salary. (During the course of this research, we learned that at least one large Midwestern hospital is guaranteeing salaries to physicians in rural communities. These individuals are not staff of the hospital, but are expected to funnel their patients to the hospital. This type of program should be carefully evaluated.) These entities would share revenues as well as expenses and would be composed of physicians of different specialties. This structure would allow the rural physician who sends patients to the group's specialists to share in subsequent physician revenues.

A financing system which pools medical expenditures makes the sharing of revenues across physician specialties much easier. The HMO concept might be adopted to incorporate satellite rural providers. Private rural physicians or providers might be able to join an HMO on a part-time basis at first, with the specific intention of switching the practice over to a capitated system after a number of years. Alternatively, rural physicians would have the incentive to reduce hospitalization rates and, at the same time, share in physician hospital-related expenditures.

Integrated systems have the potential to reduce costs and to improve the quality and availability of care to underserved populations. It would seem worthwhile to experiment with a number of integrated delivery-system models reflecting the unique characteristics of the delivery systems in different communities.

If it is not possible to link the rural practice with little or no hospitalization to a larger system, then a case can be made for continually subsidizing the efficient rural practice that cannot become self-sufficient without excessive hospitalization. Not only might it be less expensive to meet the shortfall in revenues, but also the quality of health care provided could be higher. A practice could be judged to be more efficient if the health-care costs of its patients were lower than those for comparable self-sufficient practices. It would be difficult, however, to administer a program based on this premise, particularly since making health-care expenditure estimates for each non-self-sufficient site seems prohibitively expensive. Developing a capitated system for federal beneficiaries would reward the efficient practice and is worth further exploration. The grant program described earlier for start-up and development could incorporate the capitation concept.

Peculiar Problems of Sponsored Practices

In chapter 6 we identify three factors working against the ability of sponsored rural medical practices to become self-sufficient: their orientation toward ambulatory care, their administrative structure, and their excess labor and plant capacity.

Ambulatory-Care Orientation of Sponsored Practices

The sponsored practices studied provided fewer total encounters than the unsponsored practices. In large part, the difference was due to the higher number of hospital encounters in the unsponsored practices. Providing 4,200 office visits may be a reasonable target for NHSC physicians, but this number needs to be complemented by a hospital practice or nursing-home encounters if an adequate total patient volume is to be achieved. Since hospital visits are more profitable for a practice than office visits, an additional (disproportionate) number of office visits is necessary to compensate for a negligible or nonexistent hospital practice. Increasing the number of office visits in a sparsely populated area to the necessary level may be difficult to achieve.

All this suggests that the guidelines for the NHSC program should be operationalized in terms of total encounters. If these practices were assumed to have the national average of hospital to total encounters of 25 percent, then about 1,400 hospital encounters should become the target. If these targets were reached, the practices would come close to self-sufficiency. At 4,200 visits, continuous subsidization will be required.

We also question the advisability of a practice oriented solely to ambulatory care in sparsely populated rural areas. The systems of care being developed by the federal government concentrate on ambulatory care. Such an emphasis may be more desirable for urban areas which have larger population bases and specialized services. The rural programs should be reoriented toward a comprehensive practice or systems approach that can provide a broad array of physician services, including specialty and hospital-based physician services. The types of physicians employed in the program will impact on the orientation of the practice. If physicians with only one year of internship or family-practice residency are placed in the site, the practices will have difficulty becoming comprehensive.

Having the primary-care physicians think of themselves as part of the physician community in nearby larger towns would assist in the development of comprehensive systems. In the interviews conducted, the physicians working in sponsored practices indicated that they had less contact with any knowledge of the private specialists in the nearby, larger communities. Fostering these contacts should help alleviate some of the feelings of medical isolation felt by the newly placed physicians.

The medical isolation suggested to us the development of a dual health-care system with some individuals acquiring providers in both the private and sponsored systems. Such a dual system is not efficient, nor does it ensure high-quality care. By operating in a separate medical orbit, sponsored practices reduce the likelihood of significant patient referrals to their practices. Since most rural residents are receiving care elsewhere, referrals are crucial for developing an adequate patient volume at the sponsored site. While the sponsored practices may not receive referrals, their own ambulatory-care orientation necessitates their making referrals to other private physicians in the community for secondary and tertiary care.

We suspect that one of the important reasons for the very low hospitalization rates found in some of the sponsored practices was that their patients were going elsewhere for hospital care. In this dual-system model there are subsidies for non-self-sufficient sponsored practices which are primary-care-dominated and high fees for private practices that perform lucrative hospital procedures. In an integrated system, the lucrative hospital fees could cross-subsidize some of the losses suffered in delivering primary care.

Administrative Costs and Structure

The presence of a full-time administrator, particularly in a small practice, appears to work against its becoming a self-sufficient practice. First, the administrator's salary may increase total practice costs by a similar amount. For the practices studied, other costs did not appear to be reduced because of the presence of the administrator. But, even more importantly, the administrator removes the physician from an entrepreneurial responsibility. Practice development, particularly patient volume and revenues, is largely under the control of providers. When individual patients have a choice of providers, the provider's interpersonal and medical skills become important in marketing the practice.

A successful administrative model would treat the physician as an employee. This seems most appropriate when there is no need for the physician to market the practice, but just be a member of the "production team."

The administrators' role in small practices should be reexamined. Is the administrator to manage the practice or to set the policy directions? The management role may be more efficiently taken care of by providing technical assistance to the physician and setting up systems for the physicians that can be used by an office employee. Another alternative is a part-time administrator. While this will help to reduce costs, it will not address the fundamental problem of the role the physician takes in the financial management and policy direction of the practice. Since several of the sponsored-practice physicians found themselves in conflict with their administrators in major policy matters and developed ways of going around them or neutralizing them, this suggests that salaried physicians may not be resistant to a policy shift which places them in a more financially responsible position. Certainly sponsors for these medical sites should consider instituting changes which make physicians more cognizant of the relationship between medical decisions and the financial management of the practice. A bonus program that supplements their salary, based on practice volume and net income, could be considered.

Equally important is the fact that the difficult task of practice development suggests that the retention rate of NHSC physicians in the same site is very important for practice self-sufficiency. As discussed previously, often it will take years for a rural physician to develop a practice. A change of physicians in an NHSC practice probably works to reduce the rate of patient switching into the practice. Thus, while the practice's continuity is enhanced by the consistent flow of NHSC physicians and a permanent administrator, a constant turnover of physicians may make the practice-development period much longer, or it may negate the possibility of the practice ever reaching maturity. The importance of physician turnover on practice growth needs to be assessed. It may be so important that new practices should be staffed by only those physicians with a three- or four-year commitment. Those with two years could be assigned as the second or third physician in an already developed site. The actions taken by a physician who intends to remain in a community probably contribute significantly to practice development. Sponsored physicians who have little self-interest in practice development cannot be expected to take the entrepreneurial actions necessary to develop rural practices. If self-sufficiency is a goal, then placing physicians in communities that they find attractive and reinforcing the idea that they are expected to remain there in private practice should be a priority.

If there is little potential that the physicians will become the key entrepreneur of a rural practice, then the administrator may be selected for this role.[3] An administrator, full- or part-time, may have to take on this role at a site at which there is little likelihood of the providers staying. The administrator would have to be given more responsibility over the development of the practices, not just over its day-to-day management and clerical activities. This would necessitate having a clearer line of command drawn between the administrator and the medical staff so as to permit the administrator to establish hours and scheduling. In return for the increased responsibility, the administrator should be held accountable. One way would be to link the administrator's performance with her or his income and employment.

Excess Capacity

On average, the cost per encounter of the sponsored practices was found to be considerably higher in all three major cost categories—medical, administrative, and fixed. The sponsored practices appear to be planned, constructed, and operated for the patient-volume level that would occur at practice maturity. Since the growth in a practice may take a number of years or may never materialize to the projected level because of competitors, a phased development plan for many rural practices seems advisable. With less excess capacity and lower costs, a sponsored physician may see the potential for a financially successful private practice. Unnecessarily high costs may hide this possibility.

Renovating an existing building rather than building a new one, keeping nonphysician medical personnel to a minimum, and designing a more efficient way of administering the practice are important strategies to be considered. The one input which probably should be initially designed to be in excess supply is physician time. If physicians were in excess supply, they would be more likely to take advantage of the opportunities to come into contact with prospective patients. Physicians could spend more time in the emergency room of hospitals, be more flexible in terms of meeting the health needs of their patients, and spend more time with the other physicians in the area. Physicians would have to be more responsive to the needs of the practice, for example, working longer hours on days of high patient demand. If they are inflexible in terms of their time or activities, they cause production and cost problems for the practice, because all other practice inputs must be increased to compensate for their inflexibility.

Some Concluding Comments on Sponsorship

The difficulties of beginning a new practice in a rural community reflect the need for some special assistance if the distribution of medical providers is to become less skewed. Where the intention is to have these practices become financially self-sufficient, then the practices established should emulate some of the positive characteristics of successful private practices. There are good reasons why the private practices in rural areas look and behave as they do. They have had to pass the fee-for-service market test. The sponsored models that move further away from existing private practices in terms of medical orientation, organizational structure, and provider compensation are increasing the possibility of requiring continuous support. Since dollars are limited, this need for continuous support will reduce the number of new rural practices which can be developed through federal and foundation programs.

Even if development and operating funds were not as limited, changing the rural medical-care delivery system with the development of these types of practices is a long and arduous task. The lack of a market test for these practices, the cost of continuous subsidization, and an increasing number of complaints from private providers in competition for the same patients, are likely to place these sponsored programs under exceptional legislative scrutiny. One faces the risk of jeopardizing a needed program to improve the availability of health care for rural residents for the slim chance of instituting a new method of providing medical care, that of salaried physicians oriented to primary care.

Accomplishing the necessary changes in the payment system is also a politically difficult task. The current fee-for-service payment system encourages physicians to move to larger communities, as close as possible to a hospital, and to hospitalize at high rates. Neutralizing of the distorting tendencies of the fee-for-service system on the grounds that it adversely impacts rural areas is unlikely to occur soon. Reforms which reflect the need for equitable reimbursement treatment for rural physicians would be a productive first step toward a more rational fee-for-service reimbursement system.

The rural strategy that evolves from this discussion is basically one of organization and management. It would develop practices and comprehensive medical-care delivery systems that mesh well with the fee-for-service system and existing medical environments in rural areas. The new rural programs established must be constructed so that the physician or other providers take on responsibility for a practice's development and viability. Such a system may have its beginnings in Washington with the establishment of a pool of NHSC physicians, the proper selection of sites, and the necessary level of grant support. But if it is to be successful, it must become an integral part of the local medical delivery system, at times being competitive and at other times being complementary. If it remains a foreign substance, it eventually will be rejected.

Notes

1. Other issues, such as medical isolation, must also be considered, but were beyond the scope of this book.

2. Other relevant questions that should be considered for inclusion are: How long have you been going to a practice? Where is the practice located? How satisfied are you with your current medical care?

3. Caryl Carpenter, a rural-practice administrator, pointed out in her review of the options that a multiple-site system will have a greater need for an administrator. This review was part of a presentation to the Health Staff Seminar sponsored by George Washington University, Washington, D.C., March 10, 1980.

Appendix:
A Linear Program:
Modeling the Effects
on a Rural Practice
of Varying
Reimbursement Rates
and Service Mix

In order to be able to accurately predict the success of various health-policy initiatives, it is essential to understand the financial incentives embodied in the medical reimbursement system. Here we present an illustrative analysis of the effects of these incentives on one of the practices examined, using the technique of linear programming. The practice under consideration is the solo physician, NHSC-sponsored site which is 23 miles from the nearest hospital. Detailed financial information was available on this practice from an audit of its operations, including an analysis of the practice's service mix. This detailed information allowed an empirically based model to be derived, whose static accuracy could be validated against the actual operation of the practice during the time of the research (1978). After the model is validated, several different theoretical scenarios are presented and modeled by using linear programming to determine the effects of varying reimbursement rates and service mix on practice income.

This appendix quantitatively illustrates the financial incentives embodied in the current U.S. reimbursement system and demonstrates the obstacles confronted by rural primary-care practices in their attempt to achieve self-sufficiency. The model used is based on one rural practice; however, similar incentives and obstacles are faced by many rural (and nonrural) practices, so that the conclusions presented are generalizable to many other practices as well. We demonstrate the following:

1. The hospital is an extremely important profit center for a rural practice, because it greatly contributes to revenues without adding overhead or other direct costs.
2. Raising the rural reimbursement rates to urban levels (for the practice's state) would increase the practice's gross contribution by 7.7 percent and increase the physician's net income by 26.4 percent.
3. It would be very difficult, even with an extensive hospital component, for this practice's physician to earn $30,000 or more per year without reducing the lengths of ambulatory encounters below 20 minutes,

---

This linear programming model was developed by David E. Berman and Christine E. Bishop. It is used here with permission.

substantially raising prices, or offering a more technically intensive service mix, such as adding a surgical component.

Methods

A variety of factors could be hypothesized to affect a physician's decision on whether to provide a particular service, such as a laboratory test, an X-ray, or the hospitalization of a patient. Schroeder and Showstack (1978) cite four major types of incentives which could be expected to affect a physician's resource-utilization behavior. The first, and by far the paramount, reason for most physicians is a belief that the particular service will enhance the quality of patient care. Second, physicians may order or provide services because they feel a need to document a patient's condition as a defensive measure against a possible malpractice suit. Third, physicians may provide a particular service in order to comply with patient expectations for treatment, for example, that high-quality care can be obtained only by undergoing certain technical procedures.

Finally, there are financial incentives for the physician to provide a particular mix of services. In relation to this last incentive, this discussion assumes that within the constraints of accepted and high-quality medical practice, the physician has substantial flexibility in determining his service mix and that, within these constraints, the physician will seek to maximize net income. This is not to be construed as an indictment of physicians or to say that we necessarily believe that financial gain is the strongest motivating factor behind physician's resource utilization. Clearly, if physicians wanted only to maximize their income, generally they would not locate in rural areas. What it does mean is that, from an economist's perspective, all other things being equal, an individual will seek to maximize monetary gain.

This analysis employs the technique of linear programming. Linear programming is a well-developed, popular quantitative tool of management science. Developed in 1947 as a technique for planning the diversified activities of the U.S. Air Force, it is concerned with the optimum allocation of limited resources within the constraints imposed by the problem under analysis. In broad terms, linear programming can be defined as a mathematical model that can be used to determine the best allocation of scarce resources where all the relationships among the variables can be characterized as linear.

In terms of this problem of self-sufficiency, linear programming is an appropriate analytic tool to determine if a rural medical practice can generate sufficient net income, given the constraints of accepted medical practice in a sparsely populated area. The purpose of the model is to demonstrate how this specific practice can maximize its net income within reasonable constraints and to generalize from this practice to other, similar rural practices. The solution to the model will determine the mix of ambulatory care, internal and external laboratory procedures, X-rays, hospital care, and nursing-home care that will yield maximum income for this rural practice. The model can further be adjusted to gauge the effects on income and service mix of altering certain key factors, for example, reimbursement rates or average physician time spent per ambulatory encounter.

In conducting the linear-programming analysis, three factors were varied to determine their effect on the optimal service-delivery mix and on the physician's net income: the extent of hospitalization (none, moderate, and extensive), reimbursement rates (rural and urban), and distance from the practice to the hospital (23 miles and 5 miles). (The practice's state has a rural-urban Medicare reimbursement-rate differential equal to about 7.4 percent for an average ambulatory encounter.)

The linear-programming model seeks to maximize or minimize a particular objective function subject to certain constraints. In this case, the objective function is the practice's weekly gross contribution, equal to gross collections less material costs, and the intention is to maximize it. In algebraic terms, every week the practice earns

$$(p_1 - c_1)(X_1) + (p_2 - c_2)(X_2) + \cdots$$

where X_1 = number of times per week service X_1 is provided
$\quad\ p_1$ = gross collections associated with X_1
$\quad\ c_1$ = material costs associated with X_1
$\quad\ X_2$ = number of times per week service X_2 is provided
$\quad\ p_2$ = gross collections associated with X_2
$\quad\ c_2$ = material costs associated with X_2

The constraints consist of limits on the physician's weekly time, the nurse's weekly time, limits on the number of laboratory tests and X-rays that can be reasonably performed, and limits on the number of nursing-home and hospital visits that can be conducted.

Description of the Practice

The practice is located in a Midwestern town of approximately 2,000 people. The service area is approximately 100 square miles, and this area contains about 6,000 residents. In 1977 the current physician (an osteopath) undertook the practice, replacing a retiring physician who had been in the community for forty years.

The practice provides a full range of primary-care, office-based services, including laboratory services and X-rays. However, during the period of study (1978), the practice provided no hospitalization; all patients requiring hospital services were referred to physicians in other cities where hospitals were located. Approximately 200 patients of this practice required hospitalization in 1978. In 1978 a hospital practice was planned in conjunction with the recruitment of an additional physician, a surgeon.

The practice's staff consists of one full-time family practitioner plus one nurse-receptionist and one medical-records specialist, all full-time. In addition, it employs a part-time insurance clerk. During the period of study, the practice had a very moderate net income of about $20,400 per year with the physician working 52 hours per week. The physician was on a fixed salary of $17,000, so that he had no incentive for maximizing the practice's income. (It is believed that this practice could have generated a somewhat higher net income, but that equipment and supply purchases were made in preparation for the physician entering private practice.) This is a very busy practice, which during the year of study provided just over 7,500 office encounters. During this period, the practice's collection rate was 91 percent. The physician was on a fixed salary at the time of study, but has subsequently entered private practice.

Table A-1 summarizes this practice's revenues, expenses, subsidy income, physician compensation, and retained income.

Modeling the Practice

In constructing the initial model, we assumed that the physician maximizes net income subject to resource and medical-practice constraints. The

Table A-1
Financial Overview of Modeled Practice

Revenues		*Expenses*	
Physician care	$ 70,524	Patient-care materials	$10,425
Internal labs	10,094	Internal lab materials	4,758
External labs	5,497	External lab fees	5,895
X-ray	5,945	X-ray costs	1,856
Nursing home	1,259	Nonphysician labor	8,075
		Administrative salaries	14,158
		Supplies and expenses	9,796
		Fixed expenses	17,941
Total revenues	93,319	Total expenses	72,904
Subsidy Income	17,000	Physician compensation	17,000
Revenues and subsidies	110,319	Expenses and physician compensation	89,904
	Retained Income:	$20,415	

development of the model involves quantifying these constraints and demonstrating that the resultant solution is compatible with the actual behavior of the practice. The initial objective of the model is therefore to make it fit, as closely as possible, the actual functioning of the practice.

A financial investigation of this practice shows it to be earning approximately $1,407.70 per week in gross contributions, that is, $1,866.38 per week in gross revenue, less $458.68 per week in material costs. Table A-2 presents a service-mix analysis of these contributions. Each of the figures in parentheses equals the gross collections associated with that encounter or procedure less its material costs. Note that this practice loses $0.91 for every external laboratory procedure provided.

Therefore, the objective function for this practice is the following:

$$\text{Maximize: } 7.98\,AM + 13.99NH + 2.99IL + 10.02XR - 0.91EL \qquad (A.1)$$

where AM = number of ambulatory encounters per week
     NH = number of nursing-home encounters per week
     IL   = number of internal laboratory procedures per week
     XR = number of X-rays per week, and
     EL = number of external laboratory procedures per week.

Seven constraints were identified to limit the operations of this practice. The first of these is the physician's time; he worked, during the period of study, an average of 52 hours, or 3,120 minutes, per week. It was determined that the model should first optimize the use of this physician-time endowment. It was found, partly from a time study of the physician's work pattern and partly from guidelines from the literature, that the physician spent 20 minutes for each ambulatory encounter, 50 minutes for an initial nursing-home visit (30 minutes round-trip travel time and 20 minutes for the visit), 20 minutes for subsequent nursing-home visits, and 4 minutes to read an X-ray. No significant amount of physician time was associated with conducting internal or external laboratory procedures. Therefore, the physician-time constraint is

$$20AM + 50NHI + NHB + 4XR \leq 3,120 \qquad (A.2)$$

Table A-2
Service-Mix Analysis of Modeled Practice

Collections per Encounter or Procedure		Material Costs per Encounter or Procedure		Encounters or Procedures per Week		Gross Contributions
($ 9.36	−	$1.38)	X	150.6	ambulatory encounters per week =	$1,201.99
+ (13.99	−	0)	X	1.8	nursing-home encounters per week =	25.18
+ (5.65	−	2.66)	X	35.8	internal lab procedures per week =	107.04
+ (12.70	−	13.61)	X	8.7	external lab procedures per week =	(7.92)
+ (14.57	−	4.55)	X	8.2	X-rays per week =	82.16
					Total	$1,408.25[a]

[a]Does not equal $1,407.70 because of rounding.

where, in addition to the other variables already identified,

NHI = number of initial nursing-home visits
       (first in series of visits)
NHB = number of subsequent nursing-home visits
NH = NHI + NHB

In summary, equation A.2 tells us that the sum of the times spent delivering each type of service cannot exceed the physician's total time worked per week.

The second constraint reflects a limit on the nurse's time. It was determined that the nurse spent 12.0 minutes for each ambulatory encounter, 13.8 minutes for each X-ray, and 8.0 minutes for every internal laboratory procedure conducted. In this practice the nurse worked a 40-hour, or 2,400-minute, week, so that the nurse-time constraint is

$$12.0AM + 13.8XR + 8.0IL \leq 2,400 \qquad (A.3)$$

Ancillary procedures, that is, laboratory tests and X-rays, are assigned upper constraints in this model to assume that their frequencies are within reasonable medical guidelines. Unlike other constraints, such as those on physician and nurse time, which reflect the absolute capacity of an available resource, these constraints are instead dictated by medical-practice norms. The third constraint limits the number of laboratory tests which can be conducted as a percentage of ambulatory encounters:

$$IL + EL \leq 0.231AM \qquad (A.4)$$

This constraint was derived from a service audit of another, similar rural practice. It reflects an upper limit on laboratory tests and can be roughly interpreted to mean that no more than 23 percent of those who receive ambulatory care will receive an internal or external laboratory procedure.

Because this practice loses money on every external laboratory procedure ordered, and under the assumption that these are absolutely necessary, a lower limit must be placed on external laboratory procedures. This constraint was set at the existing level of external laboratory utilization, so that the fourth constraint is

$$EL \geq 9 \qquad (A.5)$$

As with laboratory procedures, it is necessary to constrain the number of X-rays which will be conducted as a percentage of ambulatory encounters. An audit of the practice illustrated that about 6 percent of those who sought ambulatory care received X-rays, and this is roughly translated into our fifth constraint:

$$XR \leq 0.06AM \tag{A.6}$$

Finally, it was assumed that the physician would have to see a patient in the nursing home at least once per week, so that the number of initial nursing-home visits will have to be at least 1:

$$NHI \geq 1 \tag{A.7}$$

In addition, reflecting the current weekly nursing-home encounter level (1.8) and this practice's patient mix, an upper constraint on total nursing home visits was set:

$$NHI + NHB \leq 5 \tag{A.8}$$

Given the seven constraint equations, the linear paradigm seeks to maximize the objective function, which represents the practice's weekly gross contribution. The computer-generated solution to the problem is presented in table A-3, along with the actual value of the variables. The computer-generated solution generally mirrors the actual values on most of the variables; this attests to the static accuracy of the model. Actual values, however, do differ from the computed optimum values in several instances. This may be because of underlying flaws in the specification of constraints or because the physician is not using available resources to maximize net income.

For example, the rate of nursing-home visits is actually lower than the computed income-maximizing optimum. This may be because the model constraint, which allows the physician to make up to five visits each week,

Table A-3
Comparison of Computer-Generated Solution to Actual Value of Variables

Variable	Computer-Generated Solution	Actual Value
Internal laboratories (IL)	$ 25.31	$ 35.8
External laboratories (EL)	9.00	8.7
Ambulatory encounters (AM)	147.73	150.6
X-rays (XR)	8.86	8.2
Nursing-home encounters (NH)	5.00	1.8
Objective function	1,404.56	1,407.70

may be unrealistically high, so that a lower constraint might better reflect the actual ability of the physician to increase this service. Alternatively, the physician may not realize that a shift of his time from ambulatory encounters to noninitial nursing-home encounters could increase net revenue. The same holds for the internal laboratory and X-ray findings.

The computer-generated solution reveals that the shadow price of the nurse's time, that is, the marginal value of one additional minute, is 0.0, indicating that the nurse's time constraint, equation (A.3), is not binding. There is an excess capacity of nurse's time, so that the nurse could more profitably be employed on a part-time basis. Another item of interest is that the shadow price of the physician's time is $0.46, or about $27.50 per hour.

Varying the Model

Once the accuracy of the model has been verified, the model can be adjusted to observe the effects of various new assumptions on the practice's income and optimal service-delivery mix.

Using Urban Reimbursement Rates

The first variation on the model involved adjusting the objective-function coefficients by the percentage difference in the urban and rural (actual) Medicare reimbursement rates for the practice's state. The average rural reimbursement rate for an ambulatory encounter is $14.56, while the average urban rate is $15.64, an increase of 7.4 percent. Similarly, average reimbursement rates for X-rays were $23.20 for the practice's rural area and $24.00 in urban areas of this state, an increase of 3.4 percent. The objective-function coefficients, representing the gross contribution from each type of care the practice offers, were each adjusted upward to reflect this rural-urban equalization.

With these new objective-function coefficients, the basic mix of services which the practice should provide to maximize its income remains unchanged. The practice's gross contributions increased from $1,404.56 to $1,512.18 per week, an increase of $107.62, or 7.7 percent. In other words, without altering the practice's service mix, another $5,500 per year in income would be realized if its rural reimbursment rates were raised to urban levels, assuming that all reimbursements follow Medicare's pattern.

Adding a Moderate Hospital Practice

In the second variation, with the objective-function coefficients reset at rural rates, the effect of adding hospital services to the practice was modeled. The physician had found that it was too difficult to maintain a hospital practice because of the 23-mile distance between the hospital and office. Therefore, he referred all his patients who required hospitalization to urban physicians. The model is able to verify the physician's belief, namely, that a moderate level of hospital services was cost-inefficient for him to provide.

In order to add hospital services to the model, two additional constraints are added and other modifications are made to existing equations. It was assumed that if the physician were to have a hospital practice, he would always have someone in the hospital and that, on average, he would have to make the trip to the hospital five times per week. This is reflected in the following constraint:

$$HOI = 5 \qquad (A.9)$$

where HOI = number of initial hospital encounters per week (the first in any series of hospital encounters).

In addition, as with laboratory procedures, it is necessary to place an upper constraint on the amount of hospitalization a physician might reasonably do. It was determined from an analysis of the rural practices studied in this book that sponsored programs averaged 0.13 hospital encounters per ambulatory encounter, and this moderate level of hospitalization is reflected in the constraint:

$$HOB + HOI \leq 0.13AM \qquad (A.10)$$

where HOB = number of noninitial hospital encounters per week.

Adjustments were made also to constraint A.2 and to the objective function. Eighty minutes was assigned as the physician's time requirement for initial hospital encounters (HOI), reflecting a 60-minute, round-trip travel time and a 20-minute visit. HOB was assigned the value of 20 minutes as well. The objective function was expanded to include the new hospital encounters, valued at $16.54 each for both types. Note that the hospital rate is twice as great as the office-encounter rate, reflecting both the reimbursement differential and the fact that there are no fixed costs associated with hospital encounters, while there are significant fixed costs associated with office encounters. These changes are illustrated in these modified equations:

$$20AM + 50NHI + 20NHB + 4XR + 80HOI + 20HOB \leq 3{,}120 \quad (A.2a)$$

Maximize: $7.98AM + 13.99NH + 2.99IL + 10.02XR - 0.91EL$
$\qquad + 16.54HOI + 16.54HOB \qquad (A.1a)$

The computer reveals a solution where the net revenue drops from $1,404.56 to $1,380.09, a decrease of $24.47, or 1.7 percent. This indeed confirms the physician's belief. The mix of services changes as well, so that lower levels of internal laboratory procedures, X-rays, and ambulatory encounters make up for the physician's new time commitments to the hospital. This is illustrated in table A-4.

The shadow price for nurse time remains at 0.0, while the shadow price for the physician's time increases from \$0.46 to \$0.50, reflecting the increasing opportunity cost of the physician's time.

Adding an Extensive Hospital Practice

Suppose the physician could add an extensive, rather than a moderate, hospital-practice component to the services mix. Then how could he maximize income? Or, equivalently, how important could a hospitalization component be to a rural practice?

To accomplish the third variation, the same equations used in the moderate-hospitalization scenario were input into the problem with one exception. The upper constraint on the amount of total hospital encounters allowed was increased from 13 to 46 percent of ambulatory encounters. This is the rate of hospitalization used by the most hospital-intensive rural practice examined, and constraint A.10 was consequently changed to read

$$HOB + HOI \leq 0.46AM \qquad (A.10a)$$

The resultant solution is presented in table A-5. Note that internal laboratory procedures, X-rays, and ambulatory encounters continue to descend, while the physician's shadow price continues to rise. The net gain to the practice when a substantial hospital component can be added is about \$175 per week (12.5 percent), or \$9,000 per year.

Table A-4
Comparison of Variable Values for No-Hospitalization and Moderate-Hospitalization Scenarios

Variable	No Hospitalization	Moderate Hospitalization
Internal laboratories (IL)	\$ 25.13	\$ 18.21
External laboratories (EL)	9.00	9.00
Ambulatory encounters (AM)	147.73	117.78
X-rays (XR)	8.86	7.07
Nursing-home encounters (NH)	5.00	5.00
Initial hospital encounters (HOI)	0	5.00
Noninitial hospital encounters (HOB)	0	10.31
Objective function	1,404.56	1,380.09

Table A-5

Comparison of Variable Values for No-Hospitalization, Moderate-Hospitalization, and Extensive-Hospitalization Scenarios

Variable	No Hospitalization	Moderate Hospitalization	Extensive Hospitalization
Internal laboratories (IL)	$ 25.13	$ 18.21	$ 12.11
External laboratories (EL)	9.00	9.00	9.00
Ambulatory encounters	147.73	117.78	91.37
X-rays	8.86	7.07	5.48
Nursing-home encounters	5.00	5.00	5.00
Initial hospital encounters	0	5.00	5.00
Noninitial hospital encounters	0	10.31	37.03
Objective function	1,404.56	1,380.09	1,577.24
Physician's shadow price	.46	.50	.57

Other Variations

Both the extensive and moderate hospital-practice variations were further modeled with an urban-rural reimbursement adjustment. In addition to the other adjustments already mentioned, hospital-encounter income rates were increased by 12.2 percent to reflect the state's Medicare urban rate for this service. The modified equations for both scenarios are:

Moderate hospital practice with urban reimbursement rates:

Maximize:	$8.67AM + 13.99NH + 3.04IL - 0.91EL + 10.52XR$	
	$+ 18.56HOI + 18.56HOB$	(A.1b)
HOI	$= 5$	(A.9)
HOB + HOI	$\leq 0.13AM$	(A.10)

Extensive hospital practice with urban reimbursement rates (includes same modifications as above, with one change):

$$HOB + HOI \leq 0.46AM \qquad\qquad (A.10a)$$

Finally, the effect of eliminating the lengthy hospital round-trip travel was gauged. In order to establish the potential importance of hospital services to a rural practice, it was assumed that under the best conditions round-trip travel time would be 10 minutes, so that the physician's time commitment to initial hospital encounters (HOI) was reduced from 80 to 30 minutes. It was further assumed that if the practice were this close to the hospital, it would make substantial use of this resource, so that the extensive hospital-practice constraint is used. These charges are reflected:

$$20AM + 50NHI + 20NHB + 4XR + 30HOI + 20HOB \leq 3{,}120 \quad (A.2b)$$
$$HOB + HOI \leq 0.46AM \quad (A.10a)$$

This scenario is modeled with both urban and rural reimbursement rates to further ascertain their effect.

The results of all the modelings are presented in table A-6. Also included at the bottom of table A-6 are the effects of these variations on the practice's net income and on the physician's annual net income. In each of the scenarios, the physician's net income equals the practice's gross revenues less all its expenses other than the physician's salary.

Note from table A-6 that under the practice's current operating structure, merely raising the reimbursement rates to urban levels (assuming that all reimbursements follow Medicare's pattern) would increase the physician's annual net income approximately $5,350, or 26 percent. Under each hospitalization scenario, urban reimbursement rates always increase the practice's contribution without changing the optimal service-delivery mix.

Under the moderate-hospitalization scenario, the practice loses money because the physician must decrease his weekly ambulatory encounters from 147 to 117 to accommodate the added hospital-time requirements. Moderate levels of hospitalization coupled with urban reimbursement rates would nominally increase the practice's income.

Under the most optimistic scenario, that is, with extensive hospitalization rates, urban reimbursement rates, and location of the practice 5 miles from the hospital, the physician still earns only $44,315 per year delivering care 52 hours per week. Extensive hospitalization, under this scenario, adds approximately $8,600 to the physician's income; urban rates add another $7,600; locating the practice 18 miles closer to the hospital represents another $7,900.

Conclusions

Given the constraints assigned, it would be extremely difficult for this practice to greatly increase its income. Hospitalization could be important to this practice only if the use of this service were substantial to offset the travel time required. The implication from this is that for rural physicians without nearby hospitals, who also provide 20 minutes for an average ambulatory encounter, it may be difficult to make much more than $20,000 to $25,000 per year. Furthermore, it may be inefficient for solo-physician

Table A-6
Comparison of Variable Values for All Scenarios
(dollars)

Variable	Distance from Hospital (Miles): 23 (Actual) Reimbursement Rates: Rural (Actual) Degree of Hospitalization: None (Actual)	23 Urban None	23 Rural Moderate	23 Urban Moderate	23 Rural Extensive	23 Urban Extensive	5 Rural Extensive	5 Urban Extensive
Internal laboratories (IL)	25.13	25.13	18.21	18.21	12.11	12.11	14.07	14.07
External laboratories (EL)	9.00	9.00	9.00	9.00	9.00	9.00	9.00	9.00
Ambulatory encounters (AM)	147.73	147.73	117.78	117.78	91.37	91.37	99.86	99.86
X-rays (XR)	8.86	8.86	7.07	7.07	5.48	5.48	5.99	5.99
Nursing-home encounters (NH)	5.00	5.00	5.00	5.00	5.00	5.00	5.00	5.00
Initial hospital encounters (HOI)	0	0	5.00	5.00	5.00	5.00	5.00	5.00
Noninitial hospital encounters (HOB)	0	0	10.31	10.31	37.03	37.03	40.94	40.94
Objective function (gross contribution)	1,404.56	1,512.18	1,380.09	1,496.73	1,577.24	1,728.53	1,720.58	1,885.98
Changes in practice's net income: Weekly/annual	—	107/5,350	(24)/(1,200)	91/4,550	172/8,600	324/16,200	316/15,800	481/24,050
Physician's annual net income	20,265	25,615	19,015	24,865	28,865	36,465	36,065	44,315

practices to maintain hospital services if the nearest hospital is 20 or more miles away.

Moving the practice closer to a hospital (or alternatively building a hospital near the practice) would allow for substantial gains in gross contributions: $316 per week using rural rates and $481 per week using urban rates. Eliminating the bulk of the physician's travel time would allow the practice to provide more of almost all services, including ambulatory encounters, as well as expanded hospitalization. It appears that even more so than urban physicians, rural physicians may have to consider the additional financial incentive of locating their practice in proximity to a hospital.

There does not appear to be an easy way for a rural, solo-practice physician to greatly exceed an income of $30,000 per year without reducing the lengths of ambulatory and other encounters, raising prices, or providing a more technically intensive service mix, including surgery. Sensitivity analysis of our model showed that if the physician spent 17 minutes, instead of 20, providing an ambulatory encounter, the solution to the problem would change in favor of more ambulatory encounters and higher income.

The intent of this analysis is to make explicit the financial incentives embodied in the reimbursement system which confront rural medical practices.

These incentives provide important health-policy implications for improving the access to primary care in rural areas. The key to health-care delivery in rural areas may well be the way services are financed. If we are to maintain our national commitment to a more equal distribution of physicians in rural areas, then special measures must be taken. It appears that either we must be willing to assume the continued liability of supporting, through government and private grants, many rural primary-care practices beyond the two- to three-year developmental phase, or we must consider significantly altering the existing set of financial incentives.

References

Dorfman, R.; Samuelson, P.A.; and Solow, R.M. 1958. *Linear Programming and Economic Analysis.* New York: McGraw-Hill.

Heaton, H.L., 1977. *Evaluation of National Health Service Corps and Rural Health Initiative Sites.* Rockville, Md.: Department of Health, Education and Welfare, Health Services Administration, Office of Planning, Evolution and Legislation.

Kane, R.; Dean, M.; and Solomon, M. 1978. *An Overview of Rural Health Care Research: Whence and Whither.* Santa Monica, Calif.: The Rand Corporation.

Rosenblatt, R., and Moscovice, I. 1977. *The Growth and Evolution of Rural Primary Care Practice: The National Health Service Corps Ex-*

perience in the Northwest. Discussion Paper No. 5, Center for Health Services Research, University of Washington.

Schroeder, S.A., and Showstack, J.A. 1978. "Financial Incentives to Perform Medical Procedures and Laboratory Tests: Illustrative Models of Office Practice." *Medical Care* 16:289-298.

Vatter, P.A.; Bradley, S.P.; Frey, S.C.; and Jackson, B.B. 1978. *Quantitative Methods in Management.* Homewood, Ill.: Richard D. Irwin, chapter 12.

Bibliography

Aday, L., and Anderson, R., 1975. *Development of Indices of Access to Medical Care.* Ann Arbor, Mich.: Health Administration Press.

Aday, L.; Anderson, R.; and Fleming, G.V. 1980. *Health Care in the United States: Equitable for Whom?* Beverly Hills, Calif.: Sage Publications.

Ahearn, M.C. 1979. *Health Care in Rural America.* U.S. Department of Agriculture, Economics, Statistics and Cooperative Service, Agriculture Information Bulletin No. 428.

American Medical Association. 1972. *Profile of Medical Practice: 1972.* Chicago: AMA Center for Health Services Research and Development.

———. 1974. *Profile of Medical Practice: 1974.* Chicago: AMA Center for Health Services Research and Development.

———. 1976. *Physician Distribution and Medical Licensure in the U.S.: 1976.* Chicago: AMA.

Bashshur, R.; Shannon, G.W.; and Metner, C.A. 1971. "Some Ecological Differentials in the Use of Medical Services." *Health Services Research*, Spring, pp. 61-75.

Brown, D.L. 1974. "The Redistribution of Physicians and Dentists in Incorporated Places of the Upper Midwest, 1950-1970." *Rural Sociology* 39:204-223.

Burney, I.L.; Schieber, G.L.; Blaxall, M.; and Gabel, J.R. 1978. "Geographic Variation in Physicians' Fees: Payments to Physicians under Medicare and Medicaid." *Journal of the American Medical Association*, September 22, pp. 1368-1371.

Cahal, M.F. 1962. "What the Public Thinks of the Family Doctor—Folklore and Facts." *Medical Economics* 2 (February):146-147.

Carpenter, C., and Gallagher, K. 1978. "The Economic Viability of Rural Ambulatory Care Programs: An Analytic Review." Mimeographed. University Health Policy Consortium, Brandeis University.

Copp, J.H. 1976. "Diversity of Rural Society and Health Needs." In E.W. Hassinger and L.R. Whiting, eds., *Rural Health Services: Organization, Delivery and Use.* Ames: Iowa State University Press.

Cordes, S.M. 1976. "Distribution of Physician Manpower." In E.W. Hassinger and L.R. Whiting, eds., *Rural Health Services: Organization, Delivery and Use.* Ames: Iowa State University Press.

Cordes, S.M., and Lloyd, R.C. 1979. "Recent Social Science Research on Rural Health Services: A Critique and Directions for the Future." Paper presented at the AMA Conference on Rural Health, St. Paul, Minn.

Craige, B. 1977. "A Method of Analyzing a Community's Potential to Support Primary Care Services." Mimeographed. Vanderbilt University, Center for Health Services, Clinic Development Project, Nashville, Tenn.

Davis, K. 1973. "Financing Medical Care: Implications for Access to Primary Care." Paper presented at the Sun Valley Forum on National Health, June 28, 1973.

———— . 1976. "Medicaid Payments and Utilization of Medical Services by the Poor." *Inquiry* 13:122-135.

Davis, K., and Marshall, R. 1976. "Toward Better Health Care for Rural Americans." Testimony prepared for the U.S. Senate Subcommittee on Rural Development, Hearings on Rural Health Care, October 1966.

Dobson, A.; Calvin, D.; Miller, T.; Saks, T.; and Shikles, J. 1975. "An Analysis of NHSC Cost and Revenue Structures." Department of Health, Education, and Welfare, OPEL/Special Studies Working Paper No. 2.

Evans, R.G. 1974. "Supplier Induced Demand: Some Empirical Evidence and Implications." In Mark Perlman, ed., *Economics of Health and Medical Care*. New York: John Wiley & Sons, pp. 162-173.

Feldman, F.; Deitz, D.M.; Brooks, E.F. 1978. "The Financial Viability of Rural Primary Health Care Centers." Chapel Hill: University of North Carolina, Health Services Research Center.

General Accounting Office. 1978. *Progress and Problems in Improving the Availability of Primary Care Providers in Underserved Areas*. Report to the Congress by the Controller General, Washington, D.C.

Goldberg, L., and Greenberg, W. *The Health Maintenance Organization and Its Effects on Competition*. U.S. Federal Trade Commission, Bureau of Economics Staff Report. July 1977, p. 23.

Hassinger, E.W.; Hobbs, D.J.; Bishop, F.M.; and Baker, A.S. 1971. *Perception of Health Practitioners by Respondents in a Rural Area*. University of Missouri-Columbia, Agricultural Experiment Station, Research Bulletin No. 964.

Hassinger, E.W., and Hobbs, D.J. 1972. *Health Service Patterns in Rural and Urban Areas*. University of Missouri-Columbia, Agricultural Experiment Station, Research Bulletin No. 987.

———— . 1973. "The Relation of Community Context to Utilization of Health Services in a Rural Area." *Medical Care* 11:509-522.

Hassinger, E.W.; Hu, B.Y.L.; Hastings, D.V.; and McNamara, R.L. 1975. "Changes in Number and Location of Health Practitioners in a 20-County Rural Area of Missouri." *Public Health Reports* 90 (July-August):313-318.

Hassinger, E.W., and Whiting, L.R. 1976. *Rural Health Services: Organization, Delivery and Use*. Ames: Iowa State University Press.

Heaton, H.L. 1977. *Evaluation of National Health Service Corps and Rural Health Initiative Sites*. Rockville, Md.: Department of Health, Education, and Welfare, Health Services Administration, Office of Planning, Evaluation and Legislation.

Heaton, H.L.; Rhodes, J.H.; and Tindus, N.M. 1976. *Comparative Cost and Financial Analysis of Ambulatory Care Providers*. Rockville, Md.: Department of Health, Education, and Welfare, Health Services Administration.

Holland, C.D.; Durmaskin, B.I.; Donovan, C.J.; and Wolvosky, J. 1979. "West Virginia Primary Care Clinics: Development, Availability, Utilization, and Service Area Determination for 1977 and 1978," Part I. West Virginia School of Medicine, Department of Community Medicine.

Jones, J.H. 1974. "Variables Influencing Innovation and Acceptance of Changes in Health Care Delivery Systems: Jackman and Bucksport, Maine." Augusta, Me.: Medical Care Development.

Kane, R.L. 1969. "Determination of Health Care Priorities and Expectations among Rural Consumers." *Health Services Research*, Summer, pp. 142-151.

Kane, R.; Dean, J.; and Solomon, M. 1978. *An Overview of Rural Health Care Research*. Santa Monica, Calif.: The Rand Corporation.

Kane, R.L.; Olsen, D.; Wright, O.; Kasteller, J.; and Swoboda, J. 1978. "Changes in Utilization Patterns in a National Health Service Corps Community." *Medical Care* 16:828-836.

Kleinman, J.C., and Wilson, R.W. 1977. "Are Medically Underserved Areas Medically Underserved?" *Health Services Research*, Summer, pp. 147-161.

Lane, S. 1976. "Financing Rural Health Services." In E.W. Hassinger and L.R. Whiting, eds., *Rural Health Services: Organization, Delivery and Use*. Ames: Iowa State University Press.

Lee, R.C. 1979. "Designation of Health Manpower Shortage Areas for Use by Public Health Service Programs." *Public Health Reports* 94: 48-59.

Lively, C.E., and Beck, P.G. 1927. *The Rural Health Facilities of Ross County, Ohio*. Ohio Agricultural Experiment Station Bulletin 412, pp. 45-56.

Luft, H.S.; Hershey, J.C.; and Morrell, J. 1976. "Factors Affecting the Use of Physician Services in a Rural Community." *American Journal of Public Health* 66:865-871.

McKinlay, J.B. "Some Issues Associated with Migration, Health Status, and the Use of Health Services." *Journal of Chronic Disabilities*. 28: 579-592.

Marshall, R. 1976. *Health Care and Rural Development: Report and Recommendations of the Southern Rural Health Conference*. Washington: National Rural Center.

Mason, H.R. 1972. "Manpower Needs by Specialty." *Journal of the American Medical Association* 219:621-626.

Nighswander, T. 1977. "Organizational and Community Environmental Factors Associated with the Utilization of National Health Service Corps Sites." Master's thesis, University of Washington.

Paxton, H.T. 1973. "Doctor Shortage? It's Narrowing Down to Primary Care." *Medical Economics* (March 19):104-107.

Redman, E. 1973. *The Dance of Legislation*. New York: Simon and Schuster.

Reinhardt, Uwe. 1978. "Comment on the Paper 'Competition among Physicians'." In Warren Greenberg, ed., *Competition in the Health Care Sector: Past, Present, and Future*. Proceedings of a conference sponsored by the Bureau of Economics, Federal Trade Commission. Washington: Government Printing Office.

Rosenblatt, R.A., and Moscovice, I. 1978. "Establishing New Rural Family Practices: Some Lessons from a Federal Experience." *Journal of Family Practice* 7:755-763.

————. 1980. "The National Health Service Corps: Rapid Growth and Uncertain Future." *Milbank Memorial Fund Quarterly* 58, no. 2 (Spring):283-309.

Schonfeld, H.K.; Heston, J.F.; and Falk, I.S. 1972. "Number of Physicians Required for Primary Medical Care." *New England Journal of Medicine* 286:571-576.

Shannon, G.W.; Bashshur, R.L.; and Metzner, C.A. 1969. "The Concept of Distance as a Factor in Accessibility and Utilization of Health Care." *Medical Care Review* 26:143-161.

Sheps, C.G., and Bachar, M. 1980. "Rural Areas and Personal Health Services: Current Strategies." Paper prepared for the National Symposium on the Role of State and Local Governments in Relation to Personal Health Services, Chapel Hill, N.C.

Sloan, F.A.; Cromwell, J.; and Mitchell, J.B. 1978. *Private Physicians and Public Programs*. Lexington, Mass.: Lexington Books, D.C. Heath.

Sloan, F.A., and Feldman, R. 1978. "Competition among Physicians." In Warren Greenberg, ed., *Competition in the Health Care Sector: Past, Present, and Future*. Proceedings of a conference sponsored by the Bureau of Economics, Federal Trade Commission. Washington: Government Printing Office.

Stevens, C.M. 1971. "Physician Supply and National Health Care Goals." *Industrial Relations* 10:119-144.

Swearingen, C.; Schwartz, R.; and Lee, J. 1980. *Primary Health Care in Appalachia*. Cambridge, Mass.: Abt Associates.

U.S. Bureau of the Census. 1973. *Census of the Population: 1970 Volume 1: Characteristics of the Population*. Washington: GPO, pt. 1, U.S. Summary, section 1.

_____ . 1974. *Population of the United States, Trends and Prospects: 1950-1990.* Washington: GPO, Current Population Reports, series P-23, no. 49.

_____ . 1976. *Characteristics of the Population Below the Poverty Line,* no. 102, p. 60.

U.S. Department of Agriculture. 1974. *Health Services in Rural America.* Washington: Rural Development Service and Economic Research Service, Agriculture Information Bulletin No. 362.

U.S. Department of Health, Education, and Welfare. 1974. "Health Professions Student Loans." *Federal Register* 39(38):7446-7466.

_____ . 1978. *Health United States 1978.* Washington: Government Printing Office, Public Health Service, National Center for Health Statistics.

_____ . 1979. *The Health Underserved Rural Areas Program: Status Report as of December 31, 1978.* Health Services Administration, Bureau of Community Health Services. Prepared for the Senate Appropriations Committee, February 26.

Way, P.O. 1979. "Patterns in the Geographic Location of Physicians, 1968-1976." In J.C. Gaffney, ed., *Profile of Medical Practice, 1978.* Chicago: American Medical Association.

Wysong, J. 1975. "The Index of Medical Underservice: Problems in Meaning, Measurement and Use." *Health Services Research,* Summer, pp. 127-135.

Index

Index

About the Authors

Stanley S. Wallack is director of the Center for Health Policy Analysis and Research and of the University Health Policy Consortium, which is composed of Brandeis University, Boston University, and the Massachusetts Institute of Technology. Trained as an economist, he has taught at the University of Illinois at Champaign-Urbana. From 1970 to 1977, he worked on major health-policy issues in both the executive and legislative branches of the federal government. He has served as deputy assistant director for health, income assistance, and veterans affairs at the Congressional Budget Office, where he was responsible for producing legislative and budget-options papers for Senate and House committees. Dr. Wallack has published papers on several health-policy issues, including hospital-cost containment and mental health.

Sandra E. Kretz is research associate at the University Health Policy Consortium. She has been involved at the federal and local level in the design and implementation of programs in rural areas since the late 1960s. She has served as director of a ten-county program for the elderly in Mississippi. Trained as a political scientist, Dr. Kretz has taught at Boston University and has conducted research on a variety of human-services and health issues. Her doctoral research, part of which is contributed to this book, concerns demand for health care in rural areas.